Overcoming Common Problems

Coping with Life after Stroke

DR MAREENI RAYMOND

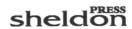

For Mum, Dad, Ramani, Paul, Tanya and Jana

First published in Great Britain in 2009

Sheldon Press
36 Causton Street
London SW1P 4ST

The author and publisher have made every effort to ensure that the external website and email addresses included in this book are correct and up to date at the time of going to press. The author and publisher are not responsible for the content, quality or continuing accessibility of the sites.

British Library Cataloguing-in-Publication Data
A catalogue record for this book is available from the British Library

ISBN 978–1–84709–058–4

1 3 5 7 9 10 8 6 4 2

Typeset by Fakenham Photosetting Ltd, Fakenham, Norfolk
Printed in Great Britain by Ashford Colour Press

Produced on paper from sustainable forests

Contents

Introduction

You may be reading this book because you have had a stroke. Perhaps you care for or are a family member of someone who has had a stroke. Or maybe your doctor told you that you had 'risk factors' for a stroke and you want to learn how to prevent it. Having a stroke is a very frightening experience. It is most often unexpected, even when you are aware of the risk, because you can't believe that a stroke could happen to you. This book explains the reasons why some people have strokes and why some people can regain some if not all of their previous independence and personality, with time.

During my first job as a junior doctor on a stroke unit, I met many people affected by stroke, both patients and their families. I remember their sense of fear and confusion. They were scared about what would happen next. In this book we will go through what happens after a stroke, in terms of what happens to the brain and the body, and what consequently happens in the hospital.

The first question everyone asks is 'Will I get better?' This is such a difficult question to answer, because a stroke affects each person differently, and some people respond to treatment better than others. One thing that suggests that people are more likely to do well after a stroke is if they engage well with their multi-disciplinary team and their rehabilitation programme.

Working on the stroke unit was unlike most other hospital environments I had experienced, simply because there were so many people on the team. The reason for this is that stroke treatment is not simply about taking tablets; instead, many different health professionals are involved. I was part of a dynamic team of doctors, nurses, physiotherapists, speech therapists, dieticians, nurses, occupational therapists and psychologists – plus many more – who helped those affected by the stroke to understand the condition better. This team is called the multidisciplinary team; its members help you to increase and eventually regain self-confidence, as well as improve and reclaim some or all of the parts of your life that at first seem completely lost. In this book we will go through the role of each member of the multidisciplinary team, how they will help you and how you can best use their specialist assistance.

Initially, after a stroke everything can feel chaotic and you may not really be aware of what is going on because of a combination of fear and the effects of the stroke itself on your self-perception. Then you end up on a ward unable to express yourself, being treated, undergoing investigations and receiving medications that you don't fully understand. Eventually you are discharged from hospital to your home with all of these new tablets to take. To make this experience easier to understand, the period just after a stroke will be talked about in detail, including tests that you may have and the medicines you may be given, both just after the stroke and when you leave hospital. We will talk about how every tablet helps you recover and how they prevent a further stroke.

Before and after a stroke your doctor will talk about preventing them. People with heart disease, high blood pressure, diabetes, high cholesterol and obesity are at risk for suffering a stroke, and having already had a stroke or heart attack will put you at greater risk for having another. That is why there are many chapters in this book about preventing stroke. You may hear it over and over again, on the TV, from your doctor or a nagging family member; perhaps you don't hear it at all, but prevention is *so important*. Modern medicine uses research to find out what things put people at greater risk for stroke, and all of the factors listed above have been found to increase the chances of having a stroke. In addition, studies have shown that people who take steps to reduce their risk factors are less likely to have another stroke or heart attack. This is why I stress over and over to my patients (and my family!) the importance of taking their health seriously and improving their lifestyle to improve their health. Lifestyle modification is a key part of prevention. That includes things like diet, smoking and exercise – all of these are factors that can be improved to reduce risk dramatically. We will also cover risk factors that you may not be aware of. For example, being of certain ethnic origin, of older age and male also increase your risk for having a stroke.

It is true that some people may have no risk factors for stroke but still have one, and this is difficult to comprehend and cope with. These are often rarer types of stroke. This book aims to cover the rare types of stroke as well as the support available to young people who have had a stroke. It often feels as though the health services are not geared to care for young people, because it is mainly older people who have strokes. This is not the case – there are many sources of support available for young people, and this is discussed in Chapter 12.

At the end of this book you should have a much better and broader understanding of what a stroke is, why it happens and how it can be prevented. You should feel more comfortable with what happened to you initially after the stroke, and you should understand better all of the tests and medicines you might experience afterward. Finally, you will understand the process of rehabilitation, both in the short term and long term, and be able to make the most of the resources available to you within and outside the health system.

Remember that you, reading this book, are also a member of the multidisciplinary team, whether you have had a stroke or are looking after someone who has. It takes a great deal of determination and motivation to get through the hard times after a stroke, and you have to give your all in order to make the best possible recovery. In reading this book you are taking a productive step toward making this time easier.

1

What is a stroke?

When you have a stroke, you may experience any number of seemingly unrelated symptoms affecting different parts of your body. For example, you may have a sudden weakness in an arm or leg, difficulty walking, problems seeing things or problems articulating words. You may have an inexplicable fall or a severe headache. Sometimes you feel absolutely fine but a family member may notice something different about you, like one side of your face drooping.

'Stroke' refers to the loss of function of part of the brain caused by a non-traumatic brain injury. The question is, how can the brain suddenly become injured out of the blue without any obvious external injury? Usually, people who have a stroke do not expect it and have no warning signs, and so it can be hard to comprehend how the brain can suddenly stop working properly.

Different parts of the brain are responsible for different functions of the body and mind. For example, certain areas are responsible for speech, vision, and movement of the right leg and of the left. If one part of the brain responsible for a certain function is injured, then this manifests in the body as a weakness or deficit in a specific area.

To put this in simpler terms, using an analogy, think of the electricity supply in a house. If one fuse is switched off, then one room's electricity is no longer being supplied and the lights don't work. In the same way, blood vessels supply oxygen to the brain, and if the blood vessels become blocked then that part of the brain stops getting the oxygen it needs to survive, and so it stops functioning. However, the following question remains – how can the blood supply to the brain be stopped, suddenly, without some kind of head injury?

Types of stroke

There are two main types of stroke. One is where the blood vessel is blocked, and this is called an 'ischaemic' stroke. The second happens when a blood vessel bursts, and blood seeps into the brain. This is called a 'haemorrhagic' stroke.

Ischaemic stroke

Joe

Joe was sitting in his garden after doing some work on the vegetable patch. He was holding a cup of tea in his right hand, but suddenly the cup slipped from his grasp. He tried to stand up to pick up the cup, but his right leg gave way as he stood up, and he found himself on the floor. He called out and his neighbour came over, called an ambulance and Joe was rushed to hospital. When he got to the hospital, he was assessed by a doctor and had a CT (computed tomograpy) brain scan, which showed that he had had an ischaemic stroke in the left side of his brain. He underwent intensive physiotherapy and managed to regain full use of his arm. When he went home he needed the support of a stick when walking.

What Joe experienced was an ischaemic stroke, which means that one of the blood vessels in his brain became blocked by a clot. This blockage in the blood vessel stopped oxygen getting to the part of the brain controlling the right arm and leg. This meant that this part of the brain became 'ischaemic', with brain cells dying because of lack of oxygen.

This process can happen to *any* blood vessel in the body. For example, when someone has a heart attack, it is because the blood supply to the heart has been blocked; therefore, no oxygen is delivered to the heart muscle, and the heart muscle cells start to die. This causes pain in the chest. Some people get pain in their legs from walking, called 'claudication' pain, caused by insufficient blood supply to the leg. There are numerous other diseases that are caused by ischaemia.

How does the blood vessel get blocked in the first place? The arteries are a type of blood vessel that carry blood to all of the tissues in the body, including the heart and lungs. As the blood courses through these arteries, little deposits can form in the arteries. Where the arteries are slightly fragile, stiff or altered already, fat and other material carried in the blood settles on these areas. They eventually build up to become plaques, called 'atheroma'. Many things contribute to the formation of this fat, such as having high cholesterol, being obese, having high blood pressure, smoking and diabetes, as well as other risk factors. These factors make the blood 'stickier' and 'thicker' and sluggish in the vessels, and they make the inside surface of the vessels more likely to allow material to attach. As the thicker blood flows through the vessels, small deposits of fat form on the inside walls of the vessels, rather like a blocked U-bend in a drain. These are called 'atheromatous plaques'. When the plaques build up, they become a larger plaque called a 'thrombus', which can entirely block the diameter of a vessel. This blockage stops blood flow at that point, which leads to ischaemia, cell death and the symptoms of a stroke.

Sometimes the thrombus can be hanging by a thread in a vessel somewhere else and become dislodged. The thrombus then floats in the bloodstream like a ticking time bomb. This type of clot is called an 'embolus' – in simple terms, it is a floating clot. If this floating clot reaches a narrowed vessel, it can become lodged and block a whole artery. If it reaches the brain blood vessels, and blocks one off, then the blood supply to part of the brain is cut off and brain tissue starts to die. This is what happens in an ischaemic stroke.

This is very important to understand, because later on in this book we will talk about how to prevent strokes, by controlling the risk factors that lead to this fatty plaque formation in the blood vessels.

You might have noticed that Joe had symptoms on his right side – his right arm and leg were weak – but the scan showed a stroke on the left side. The reason for this is that the left half of the brain controls the right arm and leg, and the right half of the brain controls the left arm and leg.

Haemorrhagic stroke

Janet

Janet had seen her doctor a few days ago because she was having headaches much of the time. Despite being on medication for her blood pressure, when it was measured at the doctor's surgery it was still quite high. Her doctor changed her medications and advised her to go to hospital immediately if she had a consistent or terrible headache. A few weeks later Janet did wake up with a terrible headache and could not get out of bed. Her boyfriend noticed that the left side of her face looked like it was drooping, and they immediately went to hospital.

The CT brain scan showed that Janet had a bleed in the right side of her brain. She was transferred to a specialist neurosurgery unit where the blood was surgically removed, and after rehabilitation her facial symptoms improved.

Haemorrhagic stroke is less common than ischaemic stroke. Around 15 per cent of strokes are haemorrhagic. They happen most commonly because a person's blood pressure is consistently high. The high blood pressure puts pressure on the vessels, and there is only so much pressure a tube can take before it bursts. It is true that the vessels are quite elastic and can stretch to accommodate increases in blood pressure – that is why your vessels don't burst when you exercise and your heart rate and blood pressure go up – but if your blood pressure is high for a long period of time then you are at risk for having a haemorrhagic stroke. The consistent high blood pressure slowly damages the delicate inside lining of the vessels, forming what we call 'arteriosclerosis' in the vessels. Arteriosclerosis is also caused by diabetes – longstanding damage caused by prolonged high blood sugar, again too much for the blood vessels to handle. The vessel walls become weakened by prolonged high blood pressure and high blood sugar. Sometimes, the high blood pressure causes formation of small aneurysms – delicate, thin-walled little outpouchings of the vessels that may burst at any time during a person's life, quite unexpectedly.

Other factors can cause bleeding into the brain but these are rarer. For example, tumours can bleed, some people have a bleeding disorder that puts them at greater risk for bleeds, and some people have malformations of the blood vessels in the brain that cause them to bleed more easily. Aneurysms can exist from birth and burst unexpectedly, presenting as a haemor-rhagic stroke.

Subarachnoid haemorrhage

Timothy

Timothy, a young father of two children, had had a difficult day at work. When he got home he admitted to his wife that he had a really terrible headache, 'like someone had hit him with a sledgehammer', but he put it all down to stress. However, within an hour Timothy could not speak properly and appeared to be very confused. He was rushed to hospital, where a CT brain scan showed that he had had a subarachnoid haem-orrhage. He was transferred to the intensive care unit for medication before being transferred to a neurosurgery unit for surgery to stop the bleeding. It took a few weeks for him to recover from the surgery and then he was discharged home.

There is another sort of bleed into the brain, called an SAH ('sub-arachnoid haemorrhage'). Only about 6 per cent of strokes are due to subarachnoid haemorrhage. Although the other kinds of strokes tend to affect older people, SAH can affect adults of all ages, including the very young. It is thought to happen because some people are born with an abnormality in their brain blood vessels that they do not know about, called a 'berry aneurysm', which is an outpouching of a brain blood vessel. If the vessel is suddenly put under pressure, it bursts at the point of the aneurysm. The subarachnoid is a thin space between the outside of the brain and the outer layer of the brain, and when the vessels in this space bleed it becomes filled with a thin layer of blood. Unfortunately, 30 per cent of these bleeds are instantly fatal. Other people have a terrible headache and signs of irritation of the brain (in particular a part of the brain called the meninges; incidentally, irritation of the meninges has the same symptoms as meningitis, such as neck stiffness and photophobia), and these people may be saved by early diagnosis, medical treatment and, eventually, surgery to stop the vessels bleeding or re-bleeding in the future.

Mini-strokes

Some strokes last for less than 24 hours. That means that the weakness or, for instance, problems with speaking or vision resolve within 24 hours. These are called TIAs ('transient ischaemic attacks'), sometimes referred to as 'mini-strokes'. The reason why the symptoms are not permanent is that, in these cases, the blood supply to the affected part of the brain is only temporarily stopped, and the blocked artery clears itself quickly. This means that the cells affected do not die, or that the sur-rounding cells compensate immediately for the ones that are lost. When the oxygen supply to the brain cells is completely suspended for a long period of time, then the cells die, and this means that the person has irreversible cell death, and a full-blown stroke is more likely. Although it is a relief to have symptoms resolve within hours or a day, TIAs are still very important because people with TIAs are much more likely to develop a full-blown stroke later, and sometimes a TIA is the only indicator that this will happen.

Other causes of stroke and strokes in younger people

As mentioned previously, the causes of strokes in young people are different from those in older people. The effects of ageing, high blood pressure, high cholesterol and the other risk factors for stroke all tend to culminate in the disease happening in people of older age. However, certain types of stroke happen in young people more often.

Haemorrhagic stroke is much more common among young people. Some 40 per cent of strokes in young people are due to haemorrhage. Some are caused by high blood pressure, leading to the formation of outpouchings or aneurysms on the blood vessels that suddenly bleed. Some people have malformations of their blood vessels in the brain from birth, which lead to high risk that these vessels will burst when these people are young.

Some 20 per cent of strokes in young people are due to sub-arachnoid haemorrhage, again because of aneurysm or vessel malformations, or rarely because of a separate illness that causes high blood pressure, for example kidney disease or hormone (endocrine) diseases.

Forty per cent of strokes in young people are due to ischaemia. In 30 per cent of these there is no obvious cause. However, the remaining 70 per cent are due to conditions that cause premature fatty plaque formation or rare diseases that cause inflammation of the arteries. Some people have genetic conditions that predispose them to strokes and other blood vessel diseases.

Some people have disorders of the blood, such as anti-phospholipid syndrome, that make the blood thicker and more likely to stick in the vessels, causing plaques or clots in the vessels. Oral contraceptives, pregnancy, alcohol and smoking can also make the blood thicker and some young people have strokes only because their body's blood is temporarily thicker because of these factors, but this is rare. Some people have inherited disorders in which the body's natural way of breaking down clots does not work properly. In some cases a tumour in the brain can present itself as a stroke, and can seem to be a stroke until the brain scan shows that there is a tumour in the brain. Taking cocaine and heroin also increase the risk for stroke, because they can increase the blood pressure in the vessels, which again puts them at increased risk for haemorrhage.

There are many rarer causes of stroke, which are more complex and cause stroke in different ways, but they have the same symptoms. Their treatment is disease specific, but rehabilitation will again be an important part of the treatment, regardless of the cause.

Will I recover?

The symptoms of stroke depend on how much and which part of the brain has been affected. They can vary from very mild weakness of one side of the body to complete weakness, difficulty speaking and swallowing, and in some cases coma or death. Some strokes are mild and resolve over a period of hours or days, whereas others are more severe and recovery takes longer. Some families want to keep their family member at home where they are more comfortable but, because of the risk for worsening symptoms in the early stages of stroke, it is advisable for the person to stay in hospital for continuous assessment and treatment. Furthermore, some strokes can progress very rapidly, resulting in worse and worse symptoms that need more intensive treatment and transfer to a specialist unit. Unfortunately, in some cases a person deteriorates so much that the discussion sadly turns to end-of-life decisions. This can be discussed with the doctors on the ward, who can give a clear and honest picture of the future.

Some people have strokes that give severe symptoms but that resolve over the course of days or weeks, with the help of rehabilitation. Still others have major strokes in which part of the brain is affected severely, and this leads to symptoms that do not completely resolve or do not resolve at all. In this kind of stroke, rehabilitation is still important to improve confidence and assess what extra help is needed to manage the disability. Some people need long-term, full-time care at home or in a care home, because the chances that rehabilitation will improve independence are poor.

In all cases, if the symptoms of stroke are recognized early, and rehabilitation and treatment are started early, then there is a better chance of optimal recovery. This is because even though brain cells can die within minutes of losing their oxygen supply, some partially affected cells can regain their function if therapy is started sooner, and surrounding cells can learn to do the job of the cells that have been lost. Many treatments for stroke depend on targeting these cells. Also, if prevention of stroke is taken into account, then the risk for having a second stroke can be reduced significantly by altering lifestyle.

2

Stroke and the brain: what you may experience

Emotional reaction to stroke

After a stroke you may feel that your personality is completely changed. You have gone through a major life event, and so it is understandable that you may feel upset, angry, frustrated or guilty. This is exacerbated by being in hospital, away from your home and your family. You may worry about who is looking after things at home and whether you will be able to lead the life you had before, do the jobs you used to do and be the person you were. Not having any definite answers about how much you will recover, if at all, can be so frightening. Imagine the person who was a plumber, an artist or a doctor, but who is now unable to use the most important tools of his trade – his hands. This can be devastating for the person who defines himself by his social, family, academic and work activities. It is so important to be sympathetic to the person, and to know about their personality and life in order to understand what they have lost.

Everyone reacts in different ways to having a stroke. My own experience of personalities on the stroke unit is that they are vastly different. One happy go lucky 65-year-old gentleman seemed not to be very upset by the stroke, and talked about wanting to get on with rehabilitation and go home. His family members were around him to encourage him every day, spurring him on and reminding him of what he had to get back home for.

Also, there are people like 68-year-old Arnold, who was determined to get back home, and gruffly dismissed any sympathy as unnecessary, having led a life in which there was no time for such things. He did well with rehabilitation. Although he dismissed his daughter's – sometimes patronizing – encouragement, and pretended not to hear kind words, there is little doubt that this helped him to get through his illness.

Another pleasant 70-year-old lady was happy to sit and chat with the medical students on the ward, with her family, with anyone, but when it came to rehabilitation she claimed that she was too tired. Speaking to her further, I discovered that she was terribly afraid of falling again and of failing to get back to normal. All of the questions and all of her worries about the future were too much for her to even start thinking about, and so she chose not to, smiling and laughing with the staff on the ward but not getting up to try to walk.

After such a significant life event, some people become anxious or depressed, and this sets them back in many ways. Sometimes treatment for these feelings is necessary. Depression and anxiety are common after a stroke, but they often go unrecognized and undiagnosed.

Top tips for ... coping with your emotions

- *Get help.* How you react to a stroke depends on so many factors and, as you can see from the examples above, much has to do with outside support – from staff, friends or family.
- *Talk.* The most important person in the equation is you – and if you have any doubts or worries, then they are bound to be a burden while you are going through treatment. It is always important to tell people about these feelings when you have them. The way that you react to the stroke will affect how motivated you are to get better.
- *Speak to your doctor.* If you are worried that your feelings are holding you back, or that you may be becoming anxious or depressed, give your doctor a call and get an appointment. Doctors can come to you or you can go to the practice or have a telephone consultation, so don't worry about not being able to see your doctor. There are so many ways in which they can consult with you.

Mobility after stroke

One of the commonest symptoms of a stroke, and what we normally think of when we hear the word 'stroke', is weakness on one side of the body. 'Hemiparesis' is partial loss of movement of one side of the body, usually an arm and a leg. 'Hemiplegia' is complete lack of movement on one side of the body. This may also be associated with a lack of sensation to light touch, pain, heat and cold, and vibrations. It is no wonder that often the idea of losing these functions is the main incentive for working hard at mobility.

As you get older, mobility should become more rather than less important. Moving around helps to prevent joint pains and stiffness and is a form of gentle exercise. Also, the more mobile you are, the more independent you are. Many older people are active in their community, and mobility helps them to maintain social, physical and psychological well being.

At first the muscles in the affected limbs become weak and floppy, but over the next few days they may become stiff. It is important to look after your skin on the affected side because if the skin breaks you may not notice and it could become infected. You can look after your skin by using moisturizer, elbow and knee pads, lapboards, headboards and foot boards to prevent injuries. If you have arm weakness some doctors and physiotherapists recommend using a sling to support the arm. This is an example of an 'orthotic', meaning a device to support the body. These are not always recommended by doctors, but the rationale for using them is that – rather than leaving your body in an abnormal position – splints and slings and other orthotics make you hold your limbs in a 'normal' posture, preventing abnormal twisted positions of limbs (spasticity). In all cases, positioning is important. Arms and legs should be kept in a safe position to prevent abnormal pulling on the joints and to encourage normal positioning of the body.

Top tips for ... improving mobility

- *Don't have a 'take it easy' attitude.* It is easy after a stroke to become dependent on others, especially because in the early stages there is an element of dependence on others that can become habitual. This can lead to a more sedentary lifestyle and decreased level of fitness. Muscle strength and stamina, as well as balance, all deteriorate, and this may lead to hazards such as falling. It can also predispose you to becoming unhappy or even depressed. Loss of physical strength has an adverse effect on social activities, such as visiting friends and family. The attitude of 'taking it easy' after a stroke reduces motivation and interest in other activities.
- *Be positive.* It is vital to be optimistic and positive when you start work on getting back to walking. The success of rehabilitation depends on your active participation and on your having a good partnership with your health care team.
- *Remember the little things.* Sadly, in some strokes the effects on mobility are too great, meaning that rehabilitation is limited and getting back to one's old level of functioning is impossible. It may be that you cannot walk or use your arm again, and this can be very difficult. However, this does not mean the end of everything. You should still play an active role in rehabilitation, because this includes assessments of what activities you *can* do and what you *can* improve on. Even if these activities seem minor, such as using equipment to answer the phone, these small things can build up to help make you more independent and lead a more fulfilling life.

Stroke and thought processing

Strokes cause obvious symptoms such as weakness on one side of the body or speech difficulty, but they can also cause more subtle problems that are only noticed later, including impaired memory, spatial awareness and concentration. These are termed 'higher' brain functions (also known as cognitive functions) and are controlled by various parts of the brain in tandem, so that a stroke in one part of the brain can subtly cause impairment.

One or more cognitive functions can be disrupted by a stroke:

- communication – both verbal and written
- spatial awareness – having a natural awareness of where your body is in relation to your immediate environment
- memory – short and long term
- concentration – ability to concentrate on a task, sometimes tested by being asked to count backward
- executive function – the ability to plan, problem solve and reason about situations
- skilled tasks – the ability to carry out skilled physical activities, such as getting dressed or making a cup of tea.

As part of your treatment, each one of your cognitive functions will be assessed, and a treatment and rehabilitation plan can be created. You can be taught a wide range of techniques that can help you to relearn disrupted cognitive functions, such as recovering communication skills through speech therapy.

Top tips for ... improving memory

- Notebooks, calendars, timetables and diaries can be used to keep up to date with daily events.
- Alarm clocks and cooking timers can help with practical tasks.
- Computer software is now available to test memory, and computer games can also help some people. Go on a course or ask someone you know to help you if you need to.
- Mnemonics can be used to trigger memories for daily tasks.
- Visual triggers can be used, such as signs and pictures around the home, to remind you of what you should be doing each day.
- First letter cueing sometimes helps you to remember; for instance, if you cannot remember the word for chair, someone saying 'ch' or 'begins with c' may help trigger the word.
- Rhymes can be a useful way to remember activities.
- Some of these may work for some people but for others they may not; a trial and error method will be attempted at first, but remember that it takes time to get into routines.
- Problem-solving games, puzzles and quizzes may also help.

There are also many methods that can be used to compensate for any loss of cognitive function, such as using memory aids or a wall planner to help plan daily tasks. Most cognitive functions will return with time and rehabilitation, but you may find that they do not fully return to their former levels.

As mentioned earlier, memory may be impaired after a stroke. In addition, several mini-strokes can result in dementia. The doctor may test your memory, usually using a series of questions that test your long-term and short-term memory and your ability to read and write.

Spatial awareness

When you look at something in a room, your brain automatically tells you the details of the object, so that you understand the object's shape, size, texture, use and relationship with the room and other objects. Many types of stroke might affect the way in which you perceive things, either directly because vision is affected, or indirectly because the part of your brain that is responsible for figuring out what something appears to be is not working properly.

Mrs Jones

Mrs Jones had had a stroke causing left-sided weakness, but she also appeared not to notice when her family sat on the left of her bed or chair. Her family became perplexed, because even if they reminded Mrs Jones that they were there she would soon appear to forget and look straight ahead of her. When she was asked to draw a clock face, she drew only the right side, failing to notice that the numbers seven to eleven had not been written down on the clock face.

This is an example of spatial neglect. It is the inability to report, respond or orient to stimuli. In addition to ignoring what is happening on one side of your body, tasks involving that side of the body become very difficult, because you must constantly remind yourself that that side of the body exists. It becomes hard to work out where objects are in relation to your body.

Tasks like eating, washing and walking around become more risky. Mrs Jones had complete neglect on one side. One way of testing this is to draw a clock face. If there is one-sided neglect, then only one half of the clock face is drawn. This means that the other side of the environment is absent, making rehabilitation much more challenging. With this ignorance of one side, you may actually have no concern about that side of your body, feeling 'comfortable' with just one side of the world. This makes daily activities more dangerous. As well as this, you may also stop attending to personal hygiene on one side of your body because it is forgotten.

For the people caring for someone with neglect, one of the key things is to understand what exactly the person cannot see so that they can alter the way in which they look after them.

Unfortunately, when there is spatial neglect as part of the symptoms of stroke, recovery from the stroke is much more difficult overall, and it has been demonstrated that there is a lower chance of significant recovery from a stroke when neglect is a symptom.

Spatial neglect and emotions

When there is spatial neglect, there may also be an emotional component to the symptoms. Emotions may not be processed in the same way that they used to be, and the triggers that used to cause emotions may not do so in the same way. Another emotion-related consequence is that the person may not have the insight to differentiate between what he or she can and cannot do.

Sometimes strokes affecting the perception part of the brain cause the person to be unable to process others' expressions and respond to them appropriately. The stroke may make the person appear sluggish and slow, and this may also be misinterpreted as being disinterested, when this is actually because of a deficit in spatial awareness. Consistently looking disinterested or bored results from a lack of variety in facial expressions.

As you can see, strokes affecting spatial awareness are complex. Because of the lack of awareness and poor memory, restoring awareness can be problematic. This is probably why people with spatial neglect have poorer outcomes in rehabilitation. The other problem is that often both the person and his or her carers do not notice that there is a problem until later after a stroke. Carers may notice that there is inattentiveness to one side of the body, or that the person only looks to one side of their body, or tilts to one side when they are seated, and this prompts referral to a doctor.

Top tips for … managing spatial awareness

Your multidisciplinary team will assess your needs and may use some of the techniques listed below to help manage spatial neglect. You, your carers and family members can do some of these yourselves.

- *Modify the environment.* This can make you more aware of the neglected side, for example moving furniture slightly into the line of vision to draw the eye that way. Keep rooms simply furnished, so there are not too many distractions to remember.
- *Eye patches.* Sometimes eye patches are used to increase use of the other eye.
- *Educating the family.* Your family and friends should understand exactly what is wrong and how they can help you, by attending a multidisciplinary team meeting or speaking to the team with your permission. Then they can learn how best to communicate with you and how to modify the environment at home to help you.
- *Simplify activities.* Break complex tasks into little stages that are more manageable.
- *Prepare for emotional changes.* Your family should understand as much as possible how the stroke may cause emotional changes.
- *Self-alerting.* Sometimes, after a stroke you may be 'hyper-aroused' as a result of a right-sided brain injury, making you much more alert and easily distractible. This is managed by simplifying the

environment and reminding yourself of your environment. This technique is called self-alerting.

- *Restrictions*. Rehabilitation can sometimes be altered to restrict movements on the unaffected side, so that you are forced to use the affected side. However, this can be hard to maintain. Encourage people to approach from the neglected side.
- *Verbal and visual stimuli.* In the case of spatial neglect therapists may use verbal and visual stimuli, such as signs around the house, to remind you of what's around you or what to do each day. They may teach caregivers words to remind you to remember your neglected side.
- *Tactile cues.* Some therapists use tactile cues, reminding you to feel around your environment to trigger memories and routine movements.
- *Speak to a specialist.* It may be that you are less able to communicate emotions after a stroke and therefore always appear to be 'fine', but only because you cannot actually express your emotions as you used to. Being able to speak to a skilled neuropsychiatrist might help you to express yourself better and communicate feelings to your loved ones.
- *Reduce risk.* People with spatial neglect have an increased risk for falls and one-sided wheelchair collisions, and may need aids to prevent them from falling out of bed and chairs. Some people may manage with these aids at home, but some need increasing care and may need to go to specialist care homes to reduce the risk for accidents and injuries.
- *Exercises and activities*. Try simple tasks first and then more complex ones. For example, try naming all of the parts of your body, or ask someone to place objects in front of you and bring them away so that you can follow them out to the side that you neglect. Do activities that use both sides of your body. Carers and family members should try to keep your brain active by engaging you in conversation, taking you out, exposing you to new ideas and asking you to be creative so that your mind is stretched to its limits!
- *Routines*. Have a set routine for dressing so that you develop a pattern to remember the left leg, then right leg, and so on. Always approach things the same way – be consistent.
- *Safety*. Make the environment safe. For example, if there are sharp corners on a nearby table on the affected side, cover them.

- *Imitate.* Ask someone to demonstrate activities first so that you can attempt to imitate him or her.
- *Repetition.* Repeat the activity over and over again to learn it.
- *Encouragement is vital.* If you are doing well, then someone should be there to encourage you, otherwise you won't know when you are being successful in a task.
- *Medications.* There are a few medications that may be used for spatial neglect, which are usually prescribed by a specialist, but so far there are few studies supporting their use.

In those who recover fully, recovery starts very early. In ten per cent of cases, spatial neglect symptoms continue for six months or longer. In those cases in which neglect persists for longer, it is more likely to become a chronic problem.

It is important to be aware that even though symptoms may seem to leave completely, there can still be some residual neglect, which means that manipulating new environments, or driving, can be dangerous. Alert family members to this so that they can look out for signs of persistent neglect.

Stroke and vision

According to one study, about 70 per cent of people with a stroke will have visual impairment. The part of the brain affected by the stroke may control certain parts of the body, like the arm and the leg, but it may also control a small part of vision. Sometimes there may be an obvious disturbance in vision, but other times the impairment can be very subtle. Vision is first assessed by the general doctor, and if there is any concern you may be referred to an eye specialist. The success of rehabilitation after a stroke can be hugely affected by a visual disturbance, so it is important to spot it early.

You may notice yourself seeing double or being more clumsy than usual. You may notice that your eyes don't move together, or someone else might point this out to you. Your eyes may hurt after reading or looking at something for a while, or you may get a headache. Sometimes the main symptom is that objects seem to move slightly. On further testing it might be that you seem to ignore one side of you (see the earlier section on spatial awareness) or you may not be able to orientate yourself in a room. When looking at something you may close the affected eye to try to improve your vision.

If communication is impaired, then it may be more difficult to recognize these signs. However, your doctor or family member might notice that you appear to be in discomfort or have difficulty doing activities of daily life. You may not be able to bring food right up to your mouth or may appear clumsy. You may hold your head to one side to improve your sight, or your eyes may dart when they look to one side (this is called 'nystagmus'). If any of these symptoms occur you should tell someone.

Douglas

Douglas, a 70-year-old grandfather who enjoyed walking, had a stroke affecting his vision. He came to notice that he could only see a small part of the room at any one time, and he often bumped into things on the right side of his body.

When his eyes were examined, the doctor found that the right half of both eyes had been affected by his stroke. This meant that he could see the left side of the room but not the right side of the room.

The problem that Douglas had is called a 'visual field defect', a very common visual problem after a stroke. This means that the field of vision is reduced because the blood supply to the part of the brain that controls vision on one side of each eye is affected. Sometimes, the visual fields will recover with time, and usually recovery is within the first months. There is no active treatment for this kind of vision impairment, but it is necessary to know what exactly is wrong with the vision so that the rest of the rehabilitation programme can be altered accordingly. Examples of steps that may be taken in patients with visual disturbance include making sure there are aids to help you manage at home, and making sure that when you are having physiotherapy attention is given to the side where the vision is poor, to make sure you learn to move safely. If the physiotherapist knows that you cannot see as well on the right

Top tips for ... managing visual disturbances

- Your doctor or an eye specialist will be able to assess what may help your vision. Consult your doctor to explain what symptoms you have, and perhaps some of the suggestions below may be used.
- Prisms such as the Fresnel Prism may be used for double vision or spatial neglect. These are thin transparent acrylic sheets attached to the person's glasses. They shift images from the 'blind spot' into the part of the visual field that is working, so that the image on the affected side is pushed to the side that works and then can be seen. Prisms can also help people with double vision to see one image. In some cases of long-term visual impairment, they can be very effective.
- Teaching you how to hold your head in certain positions may help when you have a defect in a small area of the visual field.
- Eye patches can be used alternately on each eye to manage double vision.
- Explaining to your family and carers exactly what your visual defect is makes a huge difference, by helping them to adapt the environment and be sensitive to the visual problem. Family members can also help to monitor whether vision is improving or worsening.
- If you wear glasses, you and your carers need to know when these glasses are to be used, and if there is more than one pair of glasses then they must be sure which one is for reading and which for distance use.
- Tailored eye movement exercises may help in certain types of visual problem.
- Bright lights can be used to aid reading activities.
- Remember that you must get advice from a specialist about how best to improve vision, because each particular visual problem will be managed differently.

then they will make sure that they concentrate on making any movements to the right safer. Also, when leaving the ward, it is important that visual field defects are recorded to inform the DVLA (Driver and Vehicle Licensing Agency), and to register as blind/partial sighted.

Joanna

Joanna, a 45-year-old landscape gardener, had a stroke affecting her right arm and leg. She also noticed that she had double vision, and found that her eyes hurt when she tried to read.

Some strokes cause the muscles of the eyes not to work in tandem, which causes double vision. This can make reading, looking at things and following objects very difficult, and an optometrist can help by teaching exercises to improve the strength in those muscles or by using eye patches.

Speech

When a person has a stroke that affects speech, it can make rehabilitation doubly hard. You cannot tell your family, friends and your doctor what has happened, what you are experiencing, and what you are worrying about. Speech difficulty after stroke is common, but with the help of speech therapy speech can often be partially or fully recovered.

Specific centres in the brain are responsible for understanding and producing speech. Producing speech is a complex process, involving the muscles and nerves that control breathing, articulation, the making of sounds and the projection of sounds. All of these things must occur simultaneously to vocalize words and form sentences, and so even if a small part of the speech centre is affected it can break part of the chain of speech production and render communication impossible.

Not able to speak at all ('aphasia')

Martha

Martha, a 67-year-old retired teacher, was in her kitchen cooking dinner when she noticed that she could not pick up the pepper mill in her right hand. She went to the accident and emergency department, and on her way there found that she could not speak to the ambulance crew. When they asked her questions, she could understand what they said and would nod or shake her head accordingly, but when they asked her to describe what happened she could not make any sounds come out of her mouth. She felt very frightened and upset that she could not answer even the simplest question. She felt as if everyone thought she was stupid, and became more and more frustrated.

What Martha was experiencing is called aphasia, and – as described above – it means that you can understand everything that is being said to you, but you cannot make sounds. Unfortunately, aphasia, being complete inability to produce speech, is harder to overcome in the long run. That said, some people do recover their ability to speak after working with speech therapists and with the benefit of time. It is difficult to predict how much of the brain is affected by a stroke and the degree to which the surrounding brain tissue will compensate for the loss in the brain; some recover speech well and some do not recover quite so well. Although recovery cannot be guaranteed, it is always worth bearing in mind that you may recover your speech if you work hard with speech therapy early.

Not making sense ('dysphasia')

Theresa

Theresa, a 61-year-old ex-ballet dancer, was in her study when she noticed her face felt unusual and she could not see very well out of her right eye. When she went to see her doctor, it was found that when Theresa tried to speak the words did not make any sense, even though each word was spoken perfectly. Everything she said seemed to be in the wrong order.

This is an example of dysphasia, where speech can be produced but does not make sense. This means that you understand what is said to you but you cannot express responses correctly; that is why it is known as an expressive dysphasia. Usually, there are errors in the grammar or in the order of the words.

Another type of dysphasia is caused by the part of the brain that is responsible for interpreting words. People with this disorder can speak in perfect sentences, but their response to a question may be completely unrelated. For example, Jim asks his partner 'Where did you put the sugar?', and his partner answers 'The garden looks pretty'. This is known as a receptive dysphasia – the speech that is heard makes no sense to the person who is hearing it or, if you like, 'receiving' it.

Speech sounds different ('dysarthria')

All of the previous examples describe problems that affect the centre for understanding and producing speech. Another more common speech disorder is where the words produced are completely appropriate in their content but sound odd. This includes effects such as slurred speech or high pitched, nasal speech. This happens because the muscles of the mouth and the throat are not working properly, so that speech articulation is impaired.

Dennis

Dennis, a 50-year-old businessman who had had a heart attack the previous year, was in the office when he noticed that his face felt unusual. When his partner came into the office he commented that Dennis' face was drooping to the right. When Dennis tried to speak he was slurring his words. It sounded like he had been drinking alcohol because he seemed to be mumbling. When Dennis reached the hospital he was told that he had had a stroke affecting his speech. Over the next few days, however, he found it easier to pronounce words, and over a period of months the facial droop was much more subtle, and his speech became normal.

Dennis had a stroke affecting the left side of his brain and his speech centre, and this resulted in a right facial droop, with slurred speech. The recovery from this kind of speech problem is usually good if active participation in speech therapy begins straight away. See Chapter 4, which explains more about the role played by speech therapy after a stroke.

3

What happens after a stroke?
Tests and treatments

Initially everything may feel chaotic. You may feel disorientated and afraid, and in the hubbub you may become even more confused about what is actually going on. It can be very difficult to understand all of the tests and treatments that you go through, and later remembering what happened and why can be almost impossible. This chapter explains the processes that occur in hospital after you have had a stroke, the reasons why particular tests are carried out and why certain treatments are given.

Tests after a stroke

One of the first things that will happen in hospital is a nurse checking your 'vital signs'; that is, your breathing rate, your oxygen level, your pulse, your temperature and your blood pressure. All of these tests give important clues as to how unwell you are as a result of the stroke.

These five tests will be done repeatedly to monitor how well you are and to make sure that your condition is not deteriorating. You will be seen by a doctor who asks questions about what happened before, during and after the stroke, and about previous medications and medical problems. Sometimes, speech and memory are affected by the stroke so that this information is obtained by a family member or someone else who knows you or was there when the stroke happened.

After this, the doctor examines you. This examination will include listening to the heart and lungs, to make sure there is no infection or irregular heart beat. An examination of the nervous system follows, which is a detailed examination that includes testing the eyes, the muscles of the face and the muscles of the limbs, to try to work out which part of the brain has been affected by the stroke.

Looking at the brain

To confirm where the stroke has occurred in the brain, a CT (computed tomography) scan of the brain is done. CT uses X-rays to produce detailed cross-sectional images of the body. It is a painless test in which you lie on a table inside a doughnut-shaped machine called a gantry. An X-ray tube inside the machine rotates around your body, simultaneously sending small doses of radiation through it at various angles. Different tissues in the body absorb different amounts of X-rays, and these amounts show up on the scan as different shades of black, grey and white. These scans show clearly where there is a bleed or where there is ischaemia (lack of oxygen to the brain cells causing cell damage).

Chest X-ray

A chest X-ray is also a general test done to look at the state of the heart and lungs, and it can help to rule out lung infection, chronic lung disease due to smoking, or an enlarged heart due to heart problems.

Blood tests

Blood tests can reveal whether you have a condition that might have contributed to the stroke or is making you more unwell, such as an infection. Other body systems may be checked routinely, like the liver and kidneys.

One of the blood tests will be a cholesterol test. If your cholesterol is high then drugs can be given to lower the cholesterol, and higher doses may be given to those with higher levels of cholesterol.

The neck arteries

Sometimes the doctor may listen to your neck with a stethoscope and hear a 'murmur', which suggests that the arteries in the neck are partially blocked with fatty deposit or a clot. A special scan called a carotid Doppler scan may be done to determine the extent of blockage in the artery. The reason for this test is that sometimes there is a large clot in the neck from which small clots break off and flow into the brain, causing repeated strokes. The scan shows how big the clot is and whether surgery would be appropriate. The scan is a painless one, using ultrasound. Jelly is put on the neck and an ultrasound scanner is placed over the neck to see the carotid (main neck) artery.

Ultrasound of the heart

In cases in which the heart beat is irregular or there is suspicion that a heart problem is contributing to a stroke, then an echocardiogram is done. This is also an ultrasound scan, this time with the jelly placed on the chest, and an ultrasound probe is also placed on the chest to see the internal structure of the heart and how blood is flowing within it. It can show up any clots in the heart or problems with the structure of the heart that might be making a person more likely to have strokes.

Consciousness

Severe strokes cause unconsciousness. Tests are done to see whether the reflexes are present. This gives an indication of how unconscious the person is and gives an indication of the likelihood of recovery.

Most of these tests are done in the immediate stages after a stroke, except the echocardiogram and carotid Doppler, which tend to be done after all of the initial tests have been carried out and you have been admitted to a ward. After the initial tests treatment is started; the treatments you receive will depend on the results of the scan and blood tests, and you will be admitted either to a medical or a specialist stroke ward, or to a rehabilitation unit for monitoring and treatment.

The multidisciplinary team

After a stroke you will undoubtedly meet a new person every day. For example, a nurse attends to your personal hygiene, and helps you to get dressed, to eat and to wash. There may be many nurses attending to you, and this in itself can be confusing! Your doctors will usually include a consultant specialist, a registrar (a senior doctor) and junior doctors, all of whom you will meet on their daily ward round. Each morning the doctors will assess how you are doing and decide on courses of treatment and tests necessary.

Then there are the physiotherapists, who drag you out of bed and make you do some work! Occupational therapists will find out more about you and your home situation, and try to plan a safe discharge from hospital for you, so that when you get home your house will be adapted to help you manage better.

The SALT (speech and language therapist) may meet you in the early stages too, assessing your speech and your ability to swallow.

All of these people are members of the MDT (multidisciplinary team – 'multi' means many and 'discipline' means jobs). As the name suggests, the MDT is a group of health and allied professionals who work together with you and your family to help assess you fully and create a short- and long-term management plan for you during your stay on the ward and after you leave hospital.

Each individual member of the team meets you separately to evaluate your needs and to create a report and care plan based on their assessment. These reports and plans are then presented at a MDT meeting. These meetings may be attended by you and your family.

The team

- *Consultant.* This is the most senior doctor, who oversees medical treatment.
- *House officer.* This is the most junior doctor, who may take blood tests and examine you, and prescribe medications.
- *Senior house officer and registrar.* These are the more senior doctors who make clinical assessments and start treatment if necessary.
- *Nurses.* The charge nurse oversees the whole ward, and manages the nurses and practical aspects of the ward day. Speak to them about any concerns you have. Other nurses assess your daily requirements. For example, they will consider whether you need help feeding or any other special nursing care. They are also the people who regularly check your blood pressure, pulse and so on, and look for signs of deterioration, which they can discuss with the doctors on the team.
- *Occupational therapist.* The occupational therapist makes an assessment of what practical needs you have, including help with activities of daily living, as well as your requirements to function adequately at home. He or she will assess how well you can do routine daily activities, like washing and dressing, and makes changes to the environment to make these tasks easier. They may provide walking aids and an action plan for you for when you sit up, stand up and walk.
- *SALT (speech and language therapist).* He or she will assess your speech and swallowing and teach you exercises to improve both. They also provide valuable advice on how to give food and what consistency of food to give when you are unable to swallow or speak.
- *Dietitian.* The dietitian will assess your nutrition and fluid status and how much weight you are losing or gaining. They make dietary recommendations and work with the SALT to make sure that any pureed or thickened foods provide adequate nutrition.

- *Physiotherapist.* The physiotherapist will assess your mobility and teach you exercises to move around the bed, chair and ward (see Chapter 4).
- *Clinical psychologist.* The clinical psychologist can provide useful insight into how motivated you are to recover and assess your concerns and fears. This helps to guide the other members of the MDT in their approach. As well as this, they can use therapies such as cognitive behavioural therapy or counselling to help you to work through and manage these feelings.

Together, the members of the MDT will make an action plan, reassessing and representing the information at serial MDT meetings as you progress through rehabilitation.

Medicines used in stroke

There are several different tablets that you may take as a result of having a stroke. Why are you taking them? I asked people on the stroke unit whether they knew what the medications were for, and responses varied from 'No' to 'I trust the doctors' to 'I have no idea – no one has told me anything'.

Here we will go through a few of the medications that might be prescribed and why they are given. Remember that some medicines have several different names, but all of them have an original (not brand) name that you can look up on the medicine packet.

Some medicines may be given through a drip or via a nasogastric tube at first if you can't swallow. To prevent dehydration fluids might be given through the drip. If you have high blood sugar because of diabetes, then insulin may be given through a drip to stabilize your blood sugar.

The specific medicines used in stroke depend on the type of stroke you have had – haemorrhagic or ischaemic. Before starting treatment, it is important that you have a CT brain scan, which shows what kind of stroke it is.

Medicine in a haemorrhagic (bleeding) stroke

If the stroke is due to a haemorrhage, then the main treatment is to try to prevent further bleeding. This may be by stopping any medications that might increase the likelihood of bleeding as a side effect, or by giving medication to stop the bleeding, such as fresh frozen plasma or vitamin K.

Blood pressure medicine

If the bleed is because of very high blood pressure, then medication may be given to reduce the blood pressure slowly, because lowering the blood pressure too quickly can actually make the condition worse. Medicines to lower blood pressure in the long term may be started if the cause was high blood pressure.

Blood pressure can be very high after a stroke, but this does not always mean that the high blood pressure itself caused a bleed into the brain, because even in the other type of stroke – ischaemic stroke – the blood pressure may rise.

There are many types of tablets for blood pressure control. These will be prescribed depending on what other medical conditions you have, your age, other medications you are taking, your ethnicity and how high your blood pressure is.

Sometimes blood pressure is controlled with two or three drugs because one on its own is not effective enough. Kidney function is monitored for some of these tablets, because one of their side effects may be kidney failure.

Dissolving clots

In an ischaemic stroke the medicines used are completely different from those used in bleeds because the cause is a clot. The clot is a mass that blocks the artery, which may be dissolved using blood thinning medicines such as warfarin or aspirin.

Platelets are tiny cells in the blood that make particles in the blood stick to each other, and slowly build up into a clot.

Aspirin works against platelets so that the blood is less sticky and clots are less likely to form.

Giving high doses of aspirin in the initial stages of a stroke can prevent the stroke from getting worse. It is used in heart attacks for the same reason – thinning the blood and breaking down the clot that is blocking the vessel around the heart allows better oxygen supply to the heart. Those who have had a stroke or heart attack often end up staying on aspirin in the long term, because this keeps the blood in a thinner state and less likely to form clots.

During the first 14 days after a stroke the dose of aspirin is very high; this is because the first 14 days are when the stroke is most likely to recur or worsen. After this time a lower dose is started, and this is the dose that the person will be on when they return home. Another medicine that is given with aspirin during the first 14 days is called dipyridamole, and it works in a similar way to aspirin. It is given because studies have shown that the risk for further stroke is reduced much more when both aspirin and dipyridamole are given together.

Some people are allergic to aspirin or cannot take it because they have had a stomach ulcer before, and aspirin can make people with stomach ulcers bleed. In this case a different sort of antiplatelet medication may be used, or aspirin may be used with a drug to protect the stomach at the same time, if the benefit of taking aspirin outweighs the risk of taking it.

In some cases, thrombolytics can be given very soon after the stroke. Thrombolytics are very strong blood thinning agents, which are delivered directly into the body via a drip. This is a relatively new treatment that has been shown in some studies to work well if it is given within the first three hours after a stroke, but it has an important side effect of causing bleeding. Because of this side effect, it only tends to be given in specialist centres and in very occasional cases, but it has been shown to break down clots effectively, reducing the risk for further stroke and improving the chances of regaining function and the extent of recovery.

Irregular heart beats

The reason why people have a stroke in older age can be an irregular heart beat. This is called atrial fibrillation and is diagnosed using an ECG (electrocardiogram). It may have several causes, including heart attack. The heart beats very irregularly and at random, and this makes stroke more likely. In these cases warfarin is given; this medicine is like aspirin but is much stronger, making the blood thinner by acting on a different part of the blood to make it thinner and less likely to clot. It is known as an anticoagulant. If you are taking warfarin then you need a blood test regularly to make sure that the blood has been thinned enough, and the dose may be altered depending on the blood test results. In addition, the irregular heart beat may be treated with drugs to slow down the heart or make the heart beat regular.

Cholesterol

Statins are commonly used to lower the low-density lipoprotein ('bad cholesterol') and increase the high-density lipoprotein ('good cholesterol'). Studies have shown that statins (cholesterol-lowering drugs) can reduce the chances that high-risk persons will have a stroke by a third. High cholesterol levels in the blood increase the risk that clots will form and that fatty deposits will land in the vessels. Some names that you may recognize are atorvastatin, fluvastatin, pravastatin, rosuvastatin and simvastatin, which are all essentially the same drug. Most people who take a statin have no side effects, or only minor ones. Rarely, people get muscle pains, tenderness or weakness caused by muscle inflammation. People who have liver disease should not take statins, and the tablet should be stopped if liver disease develops as a result of statins.

Goal setting

It is helpful after a stroke to have an idea of what you wish to achieve at the end of rehabilitation. With the help of the MDT, you can get an idea of what tasks and activities you want to be able to manage yourself and which with assistance, and then write these down. The MDT is the team of people who assess you after the stroke and then help you to regain your independence and previous level of functioning. It is a complicated team, including many people, *but the most important member of it is the person who has suffered the stroke – you.* Remember, the stress of having a stroke and the sad feelings that go with losing one's abilities may hinder the rehabilitation process. That is why it is important to try to work as best you can with the members of the team, and for family and friends to continue to give emotional support during the rehabilitation process.

The benefit of making a list of goals is that you are involved in making a plan and it is a good reason to meet regularly with the MDT members to evaluate how well the goals are being achieved. A time frame is established for each goal. So, many activities will have a short-term goal and a long-term goal. For example, during the next month Andrew will be able to walk to the garden with the aid of his wife. In the long term – say in three months – Andrew should be able to do so unaided.

The goals are recorded and then re-evaluated at regular intervals, to make sure that you feel a sense of achievement and recognize limitations, but have motivation to achieve realistic goals.

Top tips for ... goal setting

- Each goal should have certain features, described by the acronym SMART, which stands for Specific, Measurable, Achievable, Realistic and Timely.
- Try to let your own aims influence your goals, and discuss these

with your MDT. Some goals may be very important to you, like writing again if you are a writer. If so then these goals can be focused upon more.

- After setting goals, activities to achieve these goals are discussed and identified, and scheduled realistically with realistic deadlines.
- Some goals – in fact most of them – are not entirely achievable alone, so make sure that you know who you will need to turn to for support for each goal.
- While achieving these goals, stay positive and keep looking back at your goals to remind you of what you are aiming for.
- Congratulate yourself when you achieve a goal!

Goal setting plan

You can use Table 1 on the next page as a template to set your own goals.

How bad is my stroke?

Initially you may feel as if you will never return to normal after a stroke. The feeling of heaviness in your arm or the frustration of not being able to speak to explain your feelings to your family – all of these things may de-motivate and upset you. However, it is important to remember that some people may regain their function after a stroke. I stress the word 'some' because, as mentioned earlier, different types of stroke and different degrees of severity of stroke mean that the effects are varied. This book is mostly aimed at the person who has the possibility of regaining their usual function, or at least part of it.

Sadly, in some cases the stroke is very debilitating, so much so that it is impossible to return to normal. In these cases the person might require very high levels of care. This may include carers at home or care in a residential home. It is also important to note that some people deteriorate after their stroke, getting

Table 1 Goal setting

Short-term goal	Achieved?	Mid-term goal	Achieved?	Long-term goal	Achieved?	SMART? (If 'No' then cross it off!)	Time frame
Walk to toilet with Joanna's help	Yes	Walk to toilet with frame and Joanna supervising		Walk to toilet with frame alone		Yes	Aim to achieve long-term goal in 3 months

The table provides a template for setting your goals. An example entry is provided. Remember that 'SMART' stands for Specific, Measurable, Achievable, Realistic and Timely.

worse stroke symptoms or complications such as infections, and some of these people die. In these cases the doctors, with the rest of the ward team, will involve the family or close friends as early as possible – usually with the consent of the person who has had the stroke if this is achievable – to discuss their feelings and explain that death is a strong possibility. Talking about end-of-life decisions is a very upsetting and difficult process, and a lot of support and information should be given to help the person who has had the stroke, and the family, to cope.

Complications of stroke

Deep vein thrombosis and pulmonary embolism

When you are immobile for a long time, for example sitting on a long haul flight, in bed after an operation or after a stroke, you are at risk for developing clots in the legs or in the chest. This is because immobility leads to sluggish movement of blood in the veins, and leads to the blood being more prone to clotting, so that clots form in the legs. This is called 'deep vein thrombosis' and it causes a painful, swollen, warm leg, but sometimes the signs are more subtle. Clots in the legs may break off and flow to the chest, causing what is called a 'pulmonary embolism' – a clot in the lungs. Pulmonary embolism causes chest pain that is worse when taking a breath and shortness of breath.

To prevent these complications after a stroke, if you are at high risk for these complications (as judged by your doctor), pressure stockings on the legs may be used to encourage blood flow, and medicines to thin the blood (anticoagulants) may be given as an injection or tablets. Mobilizing early after a stroke also means that you are less likely to develop these complications.

Pneumonia

'Pneumonia' means a chest infection. Chest infections occur after stroke because your movements are limited, muscles are weak and the immune system may be lowered. The energy to cough may be less, so that particles of food may end up falling into the lungs because you are less able to swallow after the stroke, and this causes infection. Treatment is with antibiotics, and sometimes with chest physiotherapy.

Cardiac problems

Strokes can be caused by an irregular heart beat. The irregularity of the beating of the heart causes clots to form inside the heart, which then travel in the bloodstream to lodge somewhere else, causing a stroke or other medical problem. A person with a stroke is also more likely to develop heart attacks, because they have all of the risk factors for this. Many of the medicines that prevent stroke also prevent heart attacks. Irregular heart beats are managed depending on how severe they are and what type of irregularity is present.

Seizures

Sometimes the brain injury after a stroke results in epileptic seizures, which are abnormal jerky movements of the legs and arms or more subtle movements of almost any part of the body. An EEG (electroencephalogram) measures the electrical signals in the brain and helps to diagnose seizures. Sometimes medications to prevent seizures are started.

Urinary and bowel incontinence

'Incontinence' means a lack of control over when you pass urine or open your bowels. This often occurs temporarily after a stroke, and sometimes it can continue. Initially, an indwelling urinary catheter (a tube from outside to inside the bladder via the urethra, where your urine normally comes out) might be used until you are able to control when you go to the toilet. The most important point is to train to use your bladder and bowels by only allowing them to empty every two to four hours, rather than all the times that you feel the urge to go. This trains your bladder by making the sphincter muscles stronger. Pelvic floor muscle exercises can also help to strengthen the muscles that usually hold the flow of urine back; you may be asked to clench and relax your muscles down below to strengthen them. Many different medicines may be used to treat incontinence with varying success, and in extreme cases surgery may help. These options should ideally be discussed with your doctor or a specialist urologist.

Pressure sores

Sitting or lying in one position for a long time can reduce the blood and air supply to your skin, and the pressure on one part of the skin can lead to skin breakdown and, eventually, deeper tissue breakdown and infection. The most likely places that need protection are the bony prominences (hips, ankles and so on). Sores can be avoided by giving careful attention to the skin, with moisturizers and soft pillows, and most importantly avoiding pressure on one area for a prolonged period of time by regularly turning your body over, with help if necessary. This is especially important when your stroke causes immobility and you are dependent on carers for turning and moving your body.

4

Other therapies

Physiotherapy – why is it important?

One of the first questions that you and your family may ask is, 'Will I recover?' This is a very difficult question to answer. Some people have mild strokes and have difficulty regaining their independence, whereas others have very severe strokes but manage to get back to their previous level of functioning. It all depends on the extent of the stroke in the brain, how quickly medical treatment and rehabilitation take place, how effective rehabilitation is, and what sort of personality and motivation the person has.

For example, if a person starts physiotherapy early after a stroke then his or her chances of recovery should be higher, but if a person has poor motivation – because of depression or simply because of poor motivation before the stroke – then he or she is less likely to respond to rehabilitation. Another predictor of how well someone will recover is how quickly the stroke progresses and how severe the symptoms are. Those who develop unconsciousness are less likely to recover fully or even partially recover, and those who have symptoms that progress rapidly (i.e. they start off with mild weakness and quickly progress over hours to full weakness of the limbs and face with speech difficulty) are also less likely to recover. However, there are no hard and fast rules – each individual is different, and the success of rehabilitation most importantly depends on how well the team works and on how motivated the person and their family are.

At first, the muscles affected in a stroke are very floppy and weak. After a few hours or days, the muscles become very stiff, so much so that it can be difficult to move them at all. The reflexes become exaggerated. This is why early mobilization of the limbs is so important. Stretching the muscles in all the directions that they usually move in makes the limb less likely to become so stiff that it is impossible to move and so stiff that it becomes deformed (permanently stiff limbs are known as 'contractures'). Either by yourself or with the help of others, you should make an effort to move the limbs as early and as much as possible just after a stroke. If this does not happen, chronic pain and deformity can result (see Chapter 5).

Physiotherapy in bed

In the initial stages you may be limited to movements in bed only because you cannot walk or have complete paralysis on one side of your body. The physiotherapist will passively move your limbs until you can do this yourself. As early as possible, they may encourage you to get out of bed.

When in bed, positioning is so important. The MDT (multidisciplinary team) should make sure that you are always in a safe position on the bed, because you may not be able to feel your weak arm or leg, and may unknowingly cause them damage. Imagine lying in bed with your arm right under your body weight, and being unable to move it. If you are lying in an unnatural position for a long time without being able to feel that it is unnatural, the joint can become painful or even deformed in the future. When possible, you can be taught to use your unaffected arm to move the affected arm into the safest position. Pillows can be used to support limbs and make sure that they are not being dragged or pulled, so preventing long-term tissue damage.

Moving around in bed is important to avoid pressure sores.

Lying on one side for a long time puts the points of the skin touching the bed, especially the heel, the hip and the bottom, at risk for rubbing against the bed and developing sores, which can become infected. That means that your carers should ideally be changing your position at least twice a day, carefully and without pulling affected limbs and causing tissue damage.

Helping yourself to move

If your arm and leg are affected, then it can feel as if it is impossible to perform movements like sitting up, standing up, moving from one side of the bed to the other or from the bed to the chair. Also, family members may be reluctant to encourage you to move because of this weakness, but it is important to remember that in hemiplegia one side is weak and one remains strong. Try doing tasks using your left arm if you are right handed. It is hard but not impossible. If you are forced to do this over and over again, you will get better at using your left hand. This is one of the most important principles behind physiotherapy. While you must try and use the affected limbs as much as possible, you must also learn to use the unaffected limbs to help yourself use the other limbs! Some of this comes naturally, but sometimes it does not, just because the affected limbs feel like they aren't there. You need reminding that affected limbs exist and must be taught to use them safely.

Assessment of mobility

The physiotherapist starts their assessment with a detailed interview about how you used to mobilize, what your daily activities were and how you carried them out before the stroke. Then an objective assessment is carried out, watching you mobilize, carry out activities on foot and use your arms to balance and support yourself, as well as checking how much you use your hands.

This assessment includes the following:

- *Bed mobility*. How easy is it to turn to the right and the left? Can you move up and down the bed and move from lying to sitting and *vice versa*?
- *Balance*. Can you sit with or without support and can you stand with or without support?
- *Functional activity*. Can you get in and out of bed and can you move from a bed to a chair, and *vice versa*? Can you get on and off the toilet? Can you change from standing to sitting and can you get up from sitting or lying on the floor?
- *Stairs*. Can you get upstairs and downstairs?
- *Activities of daily living*. Can you wash, dress, bathe, eat, comb your hair and clean your teeth and glasses on your own?

Some people may need the assistance of one or two people to perform tasks such as eating, walking and washing. Some people need walking aids or other aids in their home. Everyone's rehabilitation outcome will be different, and even after you return home improvements may continue, resulting in fewer carers, simpler walking aids and so on. Some people, however, go home and get worse because of complications of stroke, for example having a fall, fracture or further strokes. This means that involvement with the home therapies team may need to continue. The physiotherapist may continue to monitor progress at home and in the community to track these changes and adapt the care package accordingly.

Occupational therapy

As the name suggests, occupational therapy aims to get you back to your usual 'occupations'. Occupation in this context refers to activities, occupations, skills and life roles that make you function as a whole. The occupational therapist will also try to improve your health by promoting a healthier lifestyle and better control of other medical problems. Studies have shown that occupational therapy significantly reduces the risk for deterioration after stroke and that those who participate in rehabilitation are better able to perform self-care tasks and maintain these abilities. The OT (occupational therapist) is therefore a vital member of the MDT (multidisciplinary team), and their relationship with you will be a long one, right from the moment you arrive on the ward and they begin their assessment to returning home for a home assessment. You and the OT need to have a good relationship to get to the nitty gritty of what help you will need to gain the best potential. In collaboration with the medical and nursing staff, realistic goals will be formally and continually assessed by the OT, both on the ward and at home.

Home assessment

At first everything is assessed in hospital but it is even more important to have an assessment at home, just because the home environment is the one you will be living in for the rest of your life, and that environment is very different from hospital. It may be more cluttered, furniture may be impractical and adaptations may need to be made. Simple changes may be made to make mobility easier, for example changing a low set chair to a higher chair that is easier to get in and out of. All of the assessments are carried out with an OT, because this is the person who organizes these changes.

The OT takes into account all of the following:

- medical problems
- personal habits
- physical disability
- skills of the MDT
- caregiver's needs and level of commitment
- person's needs and level of commitment

- home environment
- spatial awareness.

Functioning as a whole does not just mean getting on with the daily tasks of living. After a mother has a stroke, for example, she may feel less like a mother because she is unable to do the things that she used to do that made her *feel* like a mother. The same is true for a father, a son, a grandfather, a sibling, a friend or partner – each role may be changed in the eyes of the person after they have had a stroke, with potentially severe consequences that affect their response to rehabilitation and how they cope with the emotional aspects of the stroke.

Diane

Diane, a 45-year-old mother of two school-aged children, was always proud of her well kept home, her children and the way she looked after them. Her husband worked and she volunteered to work at the local flower shop, as well as making sure her children were well fed. She was particularly proud of her garden, for which she was solely responsible. When Diane had a stroke, her speech became slurred and her right arm became weak. During her hospital stay, she worried that her partner would not be able to cope with looking after the children on his own. When her children came to see her, she felt embarrassed that she could not speak to them properly and became quiet and withdrawn.

The OT noticed this and informed her doctor, who assessed her mental health and deemed her well enough to go home. In hospital, the OT spent time going through the daily tasks that Diane would normally do at home, such as cooking, and encouraged her to use her left hand to cook and clean with. When Diane returned home she found that she could not manage the gardening because of the weakness in her right arm, and this made her even more upset and withdrawn. Her partner encouraged her to go to the flower shop every day but she was again too embarrassed to be seen by her old friends. Her OT visited her at home and spent more time working with Diane on using her left hand to do the gardening, and tried to encourage her to pick up the phone and speak to her friends.

The OT once again contacted Diane's GP (general practitioner), with concerns about her mental state. When Diane saw the GP she admitted to feelings of guilt and worthlessness, and after many counselling sessions she was prescribed antidepressants. In the following months she regained her confidence, and this was helped by her getting better at using her left arm instead of her right, so that she was able to keep up her gardening and volunteer work.

In a case such as Diane's, the OT makes an assessment of the person after the stroke, by finding out what she used to do, what she used to enjoy, her support networks and her role in the family. The OT concentrates on helping the person to visualize what she might be able to do in future, and helps to make adaptations to the home to make this possible, for example putting in stair rails, making the kitchen safer and moving furniture in the home so that it is less cluttered. The OT can also play a wider role, as described in Diane's case, discussing worries and flagging up points of concern to the doctor.

Part of your OT's assessment will use standardized tests to assess 'activities of daily living', such as brushing your teeth, feeding yourself and combing your hair. The OT will visit your home and see how you manage daily living tasks in your usual environment and then discuss ways to improve on this. The OT will work with family members or carers to see whether they themselves can cope with looking after you, or whether other carers may be needed.

The return to previous functioning will involve repeatedly practising activities and relearning skills until your brain has become sufficiently used to the function to repeat it with less and less effort. This takes time and hard work. Unfortunately, in some cases the plateau for regaining function is low, and it is not possible for the person to be exactly the same as they were before. However, the OT should help with gaining as much independence as is possible in each case of stroke.

In some cases, the effects of a stroke are very severe and irreversible; if you are affected in this way, then sadly you may not be able to return to your own home. If this is the case, then the OT will work with both you and your family to find appropriate and useful accommodation, be it a nursing home or a rehabilitation centre. The OT will keep in contact with you and your family if there are changing needs or if there is a chance that you may need to move to different accommodation in the future. Continual assessment may help to ensure that management is adjusted according to needs.

Below are some examples of the kind of detailed advice an OT may give as part of a rehabilitation plan.

Safely washing

There are many variations in the amount of control and strength you have in your muscles, and how much help you need, so not all of these may apply to you – ask your OT to guide you.

- Have everything ready before you start your wash.
- Have the washing kit on your affected side, to encourage you to look that way.
- Make sure you are in a safe position, balanced well and with good access to the wash bowl.
- If you have difficulty standing, then aim to keep sitting down while you wash your upper half and as much of your lower half as possible.
- If you have difficulty with standing then you may need help from a carer to stand you up while you wash your lower half.
- If balance is a problem then the carer should ideally help you to keep your balance while you wash your own bottom, to preserve your dignity.
- There are several tools that may make life easier; for example, rather than putting a bar of soap on a flannel, use soap dispensers.
- Bath boards and non-slip mats can help keep the environment safe.
- Electric razors for shaving may be safer.
- You may use a suction nailbrush to clean your nails.

- You may use a suction denture brush or soak dentures in mouthwash overnight rather than using a brush and toothpaste.

Safe bathing

- Use assistance to get into and out of the bath if your OT has advised this.
- You need to be able to balance sitting and be able to lean forward safely to be able to use a bath. Ask your OT for advice.
- Use a chair to transfer yourself from the outside to inside the bath. Use your good leg to guide you into the bath; a carer may need to help you to move your affected leg into the bath and help you to swivel round in your chair, supporting your back as you move the leg into the bath, unless you can do this yourself.
- Use a non-slip bath mat.
- Use a bath board to get into and out of the bath.

Dressing

- The OT will assess how much help you need with dressing.
- If you can dress yourself, then always dress the affected side first.
- Use loose fitting and stretchy fabrics at first because they are easier to put on.
- Using Velcro or long cords attached to zip fastenings makes it easier to fasten clothes.
- Sit on the side of the bed while dressing (unless you find standing easier).
- Put clothes on the affected side to encourage you to turn that way more.
- Lay clothes on your knees first to see for yourself which arm needs to go where.
- When you are putting clothes onto your bottom half, you'll

need to lean forward a little. If you can do this, then you may be able to dress your bottom half; otherwise ask for assistance.

- Always keep one foot on the ground while you are sitting so that you maintain your balance.
- Try to learn to tie shoelaces one-handed as early as possible.
- If you need help with dressing, try to do as much as you can without putting excessive strain on your joints and limbs. If you are in pain it probably means you need assistance and re-evaluation of what movements you should be making.

Eating

- Get advice from the SALT (speech and language therapist) as to how much and how quickly to eat, and what consistency the food should be.
- Sit on an armed chair to support your arms.
- Sit close to the table.
- Use a pillow to support your back if necessary.
- Keep your feet flat on the floor with your knees and hips bent at 90 degrees.
- Keep your affected arm on your lap or stretched out in front of you on the table.
- Use a non-slip mat under the plate.
- Use a rocker knife to cut food.
- Use a plate guard if food falls off the plate.
- Use cutlery with grip handles.
- If there are visual field problems, then learn to turn the plate round to see all of the food before eating.

In the kitchen

- Use stools and wheelchairs with plates in front of them to transfer objects from one side of the kitchen to the other.
- Make sure that you have assessed every task, such as making

a cup of tea, cutting food up and so on, with your OT before
you attempt these on your own.

- To make your kitchen more user friendly, use non-slip mats,
  pan holders, buttering boards and so on.
- Use food processors to make it easier to chop foods.
- There are electric can openers and other specialized utensils;
  try them if need be.
- Use a trolley to carry items around the house.
- Put up visual reminders like signs reminding you where
  objects go and how to manage in your kitchen if you tend to
  be forgetful, or have difficulty with spatial awareness.

Speech therapy

How are words produced? You must think of the words you
wish to use and then process them, make them into a sentence,
and then use your mouth to express them. At any part of this
process, a stroke can affect your speech.

Complete loss of speech happens when the speech centre
of the brain is damaged. This means that your brain cannot
tell your mouth to say the words that you want to say, even if
you completely understand what you want to say. This can feel
very frustrating, being treated slightly differently because you
cannot produce words. Just because someone cannot speak does
not mean that they cannot understand – in fact in most cases
they can understand, and shouting will not help them feel any
better!

Speech therapy has been shown to improve outcomes in
people with speech impairment after a stroke. As with everything after a stroke, it takes hard work and patience.

The SALT (speech and language therapist) will tailor what
techniques or devices will be useful, depending on the type of
speech or communication problem. Treatment is by using techniques to increase the strength of your muscles and increase

co-ordination and efficiency of speech production. Repetition, practice, reinforcement of good speech production and breathing techniques may help. Sometimes, a device may be provided to enhance the sounds made if your speech is quiet or difficult to understand.

The most important points are to exercise speech by practice and to get positive encouragement from carers, family and friends. Educating the family on how to help you can happen at the MDT meetings or at home. Below are some of the ways your speech therapist may teach you to help improve your communication:

- picture exercises to stimulate the production of words, for instance naming objects
- repetition of phrases
- gestures, body or sign language
- word board – a device that shows single words or short phrases that a person can point to in order to communicate with others; word boards work best for people who know what they want to say but can't form the words yet themselves
- reading exercises
- writing exercises
- music therapy
- art therapy
- breathing exercises
- oral motor therapy (exercises of the mouth, lips and tongue, jaw and vocal muscles to improve strength and co-ordination).

Sometimes, rather than speech being affected, reading and writing are affected. 'Alexia' means difficulty reading and 'agraphia' means difficulty writing. Difficulty with numbers may also occur in certain types of stroke. Again, with all three, the success of regaining these abilities depends on repetition, practice and active participation in rehabilitation.

5

Pain and stroke

If you decided to sit down for a few days without moving, you would start to feel stiff. When you then tried to move your limbs, they would hurt because they have been fixed in a position for a long time. In addition, if you were to let your arm or leg go slack, unsupported, then the limb would start to ache at the joint, where the weight of the limb is being carried. For these reasons, it is common to be left with some pain after a stroke, which can further hinder attempts at rehabilitation. The mainstays of treatment are painkillers and physiotherapy, but more importantly pain can be prevented by careful rehabilitation, including positioning and physical support aids.

Joint pains

Donald

Donald had a stroke that resulted in weakness of the left arm. It took months to regain his ability to raise his left arm. He would then leave his left arm hanging at his side. Over the months he started to get severe joint pains in the shoulder.

Joint pains are common after a stroke, and this is understandable, considering the long period of time when the limbs are weak and flaccid, and the longer period of time when the limbs become stiff. As a result of not supporting the weight of your own arm, there is a strain on the shoulder, and this added weight makes the joint muscles and ligaments become worn. The wear and tear can result in inflammation or arthritis-type symptoms. Because the joint is not being moved at the shoulder, it may become stiff because of disuse, which is called 'frozen shoulder', and the pain from this condition can be very severe, especially on trying to move the joint. Slow movement of the joints allows them to 'remember' how they are supposed to move and do so more easily. It takes a long time and patience to keep doing these movements every day, but these exercises are so important in preventing the joints from 'seizing up'. If this happens then contractures (permanently deformed and painful joints and limbs) can develop. This can be extremely painful and debilitating, making rehabilitation very difficult. The simplest treatment is early movement of the limbs, and regularly practising these movements to prevent stiffening. Oral pain relief helps in some cases, but many people with shoulder pain also require injections to the shoulder to relieve the pain.

Ways to prevent stiff, painful joints

Positioning

Make sure that your limbs are always correctly positioned. If you cannot feel where your arm is, and how it should be positioned, then it is up to physiotherapists and carers to make sure there is always support for the arm, for example with a pillow while you are sitting in a chair or bed.

Care when moving

The carers should ensure that they don't pull your arm to sit you up, because this can make the inflammation and pain much worse.

Early mobilization

Early after the stroke, the joint should be moved as much as possible. If you cannot do this yourself, then physiotherapists might at first move the joint for you. Think of it like a hinge that needs to be oiled; keeping the joint still for so long makes it 'rusty' and then very difficult to move because of all the inflammation that gradually develops around the joint.

Information sharing

Let your family, friends and whoever will be caring for you know how best to position you.

Know your limits

It's tempting to try to push yourself too far when you have some weakness. Some people try to do movements that make the pain worse, because they think this will make the joint better. This is not true. Doing the movements that make the pain worse might be making the inflammation worse, because the two parts of the joint that are rubbing together rub together even more. Avoid doing over-strenuous movements that make the pain worse, and ask for advice from your physiotherapist.

Overuse pain

James

James had had a stroke that affected his right leg, but he had managed to mobilize with a stick after rehabilitation. He went to see his GP (general practitioner) because he had noticed that he had pain in his left knee, which was worrying him. After the doctor had spoken to him and examined him, he realized that the cause of the pain was that James was relying heavily on his left leg – and his left knee in particular – to support him because the right leg still had some residual weakness. When he used his stick, James leaned more toward the left and put more weight on his left leg. This led to wear and tear in the joint, and arthritis developed.

This is common in many people after a stroke or a fall and is known as 'overuse injury'. The wear and tear in the joint that is being 'overused' to compensate for weakness in the opposite joint causes inflammation of the joint, which may improve with regular painkillers, physiotherapy and, in the case of severe osteoarthritis, surgical replacement of the joint. If possible, when you use a stick try to alternate from one hand to the other.

Central post-stroke pain

Doris
Doris had had a stroke that affected her right arm and her right leg. She had complete weakness of both of these limbs, but with rehabilitation she began to get some strength and was proud to be able to write with her right hand again after six months of physiotherapy. However, when she washed her hands in cold water, she would get severe stabbing pains in her right arm, like it was being cut with a knife. The pain would settle once the water was taken away, but sometimes the pain happened for no apparent reason, when she was in bed or sitting in a chair. She realized it was the light touch of fabrics that was making the pain worse. Because the pain was so severe, she found that her confidence to do her daily exercises was getting lower, to the point that she knew she had to see a doctor to prevent her from becoming afraid of her own environment. After examining Doris' nerves, the doctor explained that these pains were due to the stroke.

The doctor explained ways to improve the pain. Because other painkillers did not work, he prescribed drugs for neuropathic pain ('neuropathic' means caused by nerves). These are low doses of the same drugs that are used to treat epilepsy. They have been shown to decrease the pain that comes from nerves and the brain. He explained that the side effects could be feeling unwell, being drowsy, having a dry mouth and getting a rash.

The second time Doris saw the doctor, the pain had improved a little but she found that there was still enough pain to impinge on her activities. The doctor gave her some advice on ways to help relieve the pain and referred her to a pain specialist. One of the things discussed was alternative therapies. Doris took up some relaxation techniques after discussion at the pain clinic, and had sessions of TENS (trans-electrical nerve stimulation), which improved her pain, and allowed her to enjoy her life again.

This type of pain is known as CPSP (central post-stroke pain), because the pain is caused by damage 'centrally' – that is, in the brain itself. One part of the brain, the thalamus, is responsible for how we sense touch, and after damage to this part of the brain, sensations that would normally be ignored are heightened and become painful. Light touch or hot and cold sensations can trigger unbearable pain in the limbs. Sometimes there is no trigger, but the pain happens anyway. It can be very debilitating and distressing. Imagine the pain you have when you have sensitive teeth – that icy pain; that is the sort of shocking pain that CPSP feels like. Five per cent of people get CPSP after a stroke. Because the pain originates from the nerves, simple painkillers like paracetamol were not helping Doris much, and neuropathic pain drugs were not completely eliminating the pain.

For many, acupuncture can help to relieve the pain. In the same way, TENS can help. This is where an electrode is placed on the skin and tiny electrical impulses are sent through the skin. These trigger the production of natural painkillers called endorphins. Visualization techniques, meditation, hypnotherapy and even counselling help some people to manage their pain.

In 20 per cent of cases CPSP gets better over a few years. In 30 per cent the pain continues but improves over the first year after the stroke.

6

Coming home

Hospital discharge

Living in a hospital is not easy, but harder still is getting back home after being in hospital for a long time. From the early stages of your admission to hospital, plans are made by the MDT (multidisciplinary team) members in preparation for hospital discharge. That is because the plan must be based on what has happened in hospital, your progress, your rehabilitation, and what adaptations at home the MDT members feel are necessary to optimize your recovery.

Jala (part 1)

Jala, an 80-year-old widow, lived in a one bedroom bungalow with a carer coming in every morning and evening to help her take her tablets, because she had trouble opening the packet of tablets. She had had a stroke that caused weakness in her right leg and right arm. Her house was visited by the OT (occupational therapist) while she was in hospital and was noted to be quite cluttered. The step to get to the front door was also a little slanted. When Jala came home for an assessment of her mobility at home, one of the main problems was that she could not get around with the stick she had learnt to walk with, because of the clutter. In addition, when she went to the bathroom she found it very difficult to balance while getting into and out of the bath, or sitting on the toilet seat.

The OT arranged for a new step to be fitted in front of the house, and fixed bath and toilet handrails to make getting into and out of the bath easier, with a non-slip bath mat in the bath. Carer visits were increased to three times a day, to make sure that Jala was managing with washing, dressing and mobilizing. (This was later reduced to carer visits twice a day, because Jala had no problems making food and getting around her house over the following weeks.)

While these adjustments were taking place and Jala was well enough to be discharged from hospital, she stayed in a residential home for two days before going to her bungalow again.

Naturally, it takes time to organize a safe discharge, and sometimes a too speedy discharge from the ward can lead to problems such as falls and fractures, depression and many other conditions. It is therefore best to be safe when it comes to planning the hospital discharge. That is why Jala stayed in a residential home – a safe environment that is not a hospital – until her home was prepared.

What influences the outcome of hospital discharge?

Some of the factors that can influence outcomes after hospital discharge are as follows:

- pre-stroke medical problems
- pre-stroke level of function
- impairment as a result of stroke
- family support
- age
- psychosocial factors (e.g. difficult relationships, lack of support, depression and anxiety)
- medical complications.

Many people already have some disability before their stroke, so full recovery is challenging. People with many medical problems are less likely to be able to resume their normal activities unless they have a great deal of support.

Other factors that have been found to influence outcomes after a stroke are having a better education, being female, having a good pre-stroke level of functioning and having a spouse. All of these factors increase the likelihood of having a more fulfilled social life on returning home after a stroke, and there are many theories as to why this might be so.

The community

What is the community? This depends on where you live. In the inner city there may be a neighbour who checks on you every so often, or a dance class in town that provides a social network. In rural areas perhaps the community really is the people who live around you and who you meet on your visits to the shops. Whatever community is to you, the MDT aims to reintegrate you back into that community. Some people are not involved in any sort of community activity, be it shopping, walking or socializing in the park, and in these cases coming to hospital may bring up the discussion about how much you would like to be more involved in the community. Depending on your age and level of functioning, as well as your preferences of course, there are several ways to reintegrate into the community.

Jala (part 2)

While in hospital, Jala visited her home close to the time of discharge. The OT walked to town with her to see what sort of things Jala normally did at home. This included daily shopping trips and popping to the post office. The OT helped Jala to carry her shopping back because Jala walked with a stick and found carrying the bags too difficult. After her hospital discharge, Jala at first felt fearful to walk around her town on her own, and so the OT suggested that her carer help her to walk to the shops in the morning after breakfast and assist her with her shopping. She managed to walk to the shops and back with the help of her carer. After a few weeks Jala managed to go into the town on her own to do manageable tasks like going to the post office, where she often bumped into old friends. She bumped into a friend who invited her to join the church whist group. Jala took up the offer and walked every Saturday to church to play whist.

If you are to get used to living in the community and taking part in social activities, then this must happen early in rehabilitation. The OT might introduce you to local community centres and other activity groups that are of interest to you while you are still in hospital. By the time you are discharged you are more likely to have become comfortable with a community activity and choose to maintain that activity after the discharge. As well as this, routine activities such as getting to the bank, the post office and the shops can be practised before the official discharge from hospital. Community therapists will often continue to provide input when you go home to avoid setbacks that may occur on going from the hospital environment to the 'real' world.

Other services may be provided after hospital discharge, temporarily or permanently, such as meals on wheels and carers, counsellors, volunteer befriending services and more. There are day centres that provide activities for people, and there are charity organizations for people with many different medical and social circumstances, which are worth investigating if available. For people caring for a family member, and who need to go on holiday or have a break from their caring duties for personal reasons, there are sometimes respite homes available where a person can stay for a few days and take part in a social programme. You can find out more about what is available from your local council or your GP (general practitioner), or use the internet to research activities in the area.

Leisure

Some people like the idea of taking up a hobby to keep active and lead a fuller life; others do not like the idea, and it is left up to the individual to decide what level of activity is appropriate for them. Many outdoor and indoor activities can now be adapted for a person with a disability – even horse riding! It is therefore worth looking into what opportunities are available in the local area if you have an interest in doing something new.

Ask yourself the following questions.

- What did I enjoy doing? It doesn't have to be something exciting – even housework is a leisure activity for some!
- Can I do the same things but at a slower pace?

- Alternatively, should I try something new, because I can't do what I used to?
- Do I want to do activities on my own, or do I want to be part of a social group?
- Do I want to spend more time outdoors?
- Do I enjoy indoor activities, like watching TV, reading and cooking?
- Do I need new spectacles or a hearing aid to make a task easier?
- Do I know someone who might want to take up this interest with me?
- Are there any local agencies or voluntary organizations that could help me?
- Can I use the internet or the telephone directory to find out what's going on around my area?

Sometimes you need the support of a friend or family member to gain courage to take up an activity. Apprehension or nervousness can be overcome by going to support groups or other groups, where people meet each other and make friends, so that they can take up an activity like arts and crafts together. Of course, this is easier said than done, and sometimes there are too many barriers to this sort of socializing or group activity. There are several activities and hobbies that are solitary and just as fun for many.

Take reading for example. Immersing yourself in a good story or learning something new through reading is a fantastic hobby, whether it be reading the daily newspaper or books. There are large print books and audio tapes for those who have reading difficulty. Other hobbies such as watching TV, knitting and crosswords are equally good. One gentleman I met on the stroke unit later learnt how to use a computer at his local community centre, where they provided a programme to help improve reading and arithmetic and keep the mind on its toes!

Getting back to work

Many people are employed at the time of their stroke, and the thought of not going back to work can either be a positive or a negative one! It's fair enough that many people want to resume their usual duties after a stroke, and that is possible in many cases. It is great to feel motivated and to love your job, and this is something that should be promoted, because it is part of regaining your old life. However, sometimes the stroke is debilitating enough to stop you from doing your old job. Then what do you do?

Talk to your employer

Get advice from your employer if you feel that he or she is approachable and supportive or if you need some advice about how your job could be adapted for you. If an employer is supportive, then returning to work is much more likely to be successful. There may be certain tasks that need more physical work or stamina, and it is worth having a realistic discussion with your employer about what level of activity you can get back to.

Talk to a specialist

Sometimes your employer cannot take you back. Get in touch with your union or occupational health department to get advice on your rights. At the job centre a disability employment advisor can help to assess your ability to work. They can liaise with your employer to find out whether it is possible for you to work there, with some assistance or special equipment. Remember to get advice from organizations such as The Stroke Association with experience in these matters.

Consider your options

Many people decide to change jobs or to do voluntary work, according to what they feel they can do, and this works well for many. Ask yourself the following questions:

- Is it important that I get paid in my work?
- Would voluntary work be fulfilling for me?
- Would it help me to work, as part of my old routine?
- Would it help me to do something productive, like working?
- Is it important to me to maintain my previous role?
- Do I need to go to work to help motivate me in other things?
- Do I need to be challenged?

Don't be put off

Some people are put off by their disability, feeling embarrassed or sad about it and not being encouraged by family and friends, leading them to stop working or to take up a different, more manageable job. Try not to let your fear get in the way of doing what you want to do, and always make an effort to talk to someone – a friend, family member, GP or counsellor – about these feelings and how to overcome them.

Have a discussion with your occupational therapist

The OT will help you to establish realistic goals when it comes to getting back to work. Many jobs may need to be broken up into more easily handled small jobs.

Volunteer

Sometimes it is not possible to get back to work, and voluntary work may be more appropriate. Many people I have met have had exciting opportunities brought to them after a stroke through voluntary work.

Driving

After a stroke the official line is that you must not drive for at least one month. After this driving is permitted only if it is deemed safe, and this is determined by an assessment conducted by the OT. Ultimately, it is the GP who decides whether you are fit to drive or not. The GP fills in a form confirming medical problems, and this is reviewed by the DVLA (Driver and Vehicle Licensing Agency), which will decide whether to grant a licence.

Sexuality and stroke

The thought of having sex after a stroke may be daunting. Many people find it difficult to resume sexual activity, and that is because of tiredness from the increased effort to do things, as well as embarrassment, and worry about not being able to get into sexual positions. Some feel that after a stroke it is dangerous to have sex, but this is not true.

In addition, sexual intercourse may be difficult because of being overweight, having diabetes with nervous system involvement, and being on multiple medications, some of which have the side effect of making sex more difficult. Although stroke *per se* does not alter libido, the effects of having these risk factors already, as well as reduced confidence after a stroke and the complications of stroke, can all make getting back to sexual activity very frustrating and difficult. Sex is not often talked about as part of rehabilitation, despite it being an important part of many people's lives before they have a stroke and equally so afterward.

There are many ways that you can try to overcome difficulties, depending on what is holding you back. Examples include the following.

- *Talking.* Talk to your partner about your feelings, and your concerns, and try to work together on solutions. Talk to your GP if you worry that your medications may be affecting your sex life, or if you feel that counselling might help.
- *Humour.* Relax with your partner, laugh and do things that you enjoy together, to increase intimacy.
- *Try new things in bed.* Spend more time on foreplay and intimacy before sexual intercourse.

- *Hygiene*. Try to maintain personal hygiene.
- *Plan*. If you are having trouble making time for sex, plan for it. In addition, take into account what you need to prepare for in practical terms; for example, if you are worried about incontinence, then make sure you plan ahead by going to the toilet before having sex.
- *Relaxation*. Try massage, aromatherapy or taking baths together to relax together before sex.
- *Try different positions*. If weakness makes certain positions difficult, then talk to your partner about trying different positions.

The Stroke Association has a leaflet about sex after a stroke, which is available on the internet (<http://www.stroke.org.uk/information/our_publications/factsheets/31_sex_after.html>) and ideally should be given to all persons after they have had a stroke.

7

How family and friends can help

This section of the book is directed at family members, friends and carers, although the person who has had a stroke will also benefit from reading it.

Communicating with a person who has had a stroke

There have been many accounts of how a person feels after having suffered some illness or disability, and how it can feel as though he or she is treated differently after such an event. That is because it's true – people do treat someone differently when he or she is ill, perhaps in a well meaning way but sometimes not quite the right way. One account by a man who had become visually impaired described how he felt that people touched him less after he became visually impaired, perhaps because they felt uncomfortable.

It is understandable that you may be afraid of illness and of upsetting someone who has become unwell. It's hard to know how he or she might respond and how best to make that person feel better. There are no set rules – everyone is different, and everyone's reaction to stroke will be different.

For some people the simple act of hand holding, or giving them a hug or a kiss can make them feel better – this is probably even more so when that someone is ill. Of course, some people gruffly deal with the illness, wanting to 'bear up' and 'be a man', and in those sorts of personalities support is provided in a different way, but these people still need the touch of others like they did before they became unwell.

Dignity is very important. In the hospital, sadly, it can feel like dignity is lost completely, with the person having little privacy in the hospital bed, being manhandled by strangers and depending on others for washing, dressing and toileting. However, the manner in which these things are done can maintain a person's dignity.

- Talking clearly to the person, in the same way that you would before he or she became ill, is a simple way to maintain dignity.
- In hospital or in a residential home, or even in the home, a person who has suffered a stroke may find it difficult to keep the 'order' maintained before he or she had the stroke. By simply asking a few questions about a person's previous lifestyle and habits, and about preferences regarding how things are arranged, dignity and pre-stroke levels of happiness can be achieved.
- Communication after an illness is often hindered by physical barriers. Someone who is sitting in a chair or bed with decreased vision or hearing will appreciate it if you notice these things and adapt your communication accordingly. For example, ensuring that you are on the same level as the person, so that he or she can see your face, eyes and lips, can improve communication.
- Make sure there is no background noise and ensure privacy in a conversation; this results in comfortable communication.
- You should check that visual aids and hearing aids are working! Shouting at a hearing impaired person or turning the hearing aid up can just make it harder to hear. The person should be asked about what level of sound is best for him or her to avoid embarrassing and undignified conversations.

Being a carer

Mutual agreement between the person who has suffered a stroke and his or her partner, other family members or friends may result in a non-professional being the main carer – but that person is often an expert in the person who has had a stroke! If you decide to care for a family member or friend, the responsibility is great and the job is not easy. As well as physical work, such as helping a person to walk around or sit up, there are the added emotional demands of someone whose personality may have changed, and the emotional strain of seeing a loved one in a very different light. It is not surprising that carers, whether they are provided by the Government or privately, or whether they know the person independently, are under a lot of pressure when looking after someone.

After a stroke, it is worth the person entering into a discussion with family members about what sort of care package he or she wants and whether a family member would be preferable as the main carer. The benefits of a carer within the family are many, because this person knows their affected family member well and can also handle the financial side of things, as well as being a dedicated co-ordinator of other services from home. However, it may mean that the carer has to give up a job, and may need to go through training, depending on what the social worker feels is necessary.

When you are making a decision about whether to be a carer, consider the following questions.

- Will you live with the person who has had a stroke?
- Is the house appropriately set out? For example, is there a downstairs toilet if the person cannot get upstairs?
- Can you both cope financially?
- Are there other people in the family who may want to be involved in this decision?
- Are there stairs in the house?
- Are there enough toilets?
- Can the OT suggest adaptations to the house?
- Will you be able to cope with caring responsibilities?
- How can you and the person who has had a stroke continue to play your roles in the family?

- Do you need special training?
- Do you understand the medical conditions?
- What help will you receive?

A carer can become ill and tired, and decide that they cannot care for someone else any more. This is hard to admit to in an attempt to 'stay strong' and support your loved one, but it is not worth pushing yourself so much that you are exhausted. You can always get extra help, or allow professional carers to take over or support your role.

Below is some general advice on how to cope with being a carer. (See *The Complete Carer's Guide* by Bridget McCall, also published by Sheldon Press.)

Positivity

Rehabilitation can be a slow and frustrating process, and there will be periods when it appears that little progress has been made. Encouraging and praising any progress, no matter how small it may appear, can help motivate someone who has had a stroke to achieve his or her long-term goals.

Ask for help

There are a wide range of support services and resources available for people who are recovering from strokes, and their families and carers. These range from equipment that can help with mobility to psychological support for carers and families. The hospital staff involved with the rehabilitation process will be able to provide advice and relevant contact information.

Make time for yourself

If you are caring for someone who has had a stroke, it is important not to neglect your own physical and psychological well being. Socializing with friends or pursuing leisure interests will help you to cope better with the situation. Recognizing when you are not having enough 'you time' can be near impossible when you are in the situation itself, so make sure that you talk to others about what you are feeling and take a moment every day to evaluate what you have done during the day for yourself.

8

Nutrition and stroke

Diet is important in many ways when it comes to prevention of and recovery from a stroke. We already know that diet can influence the chances of having a stroke, so an understanding of what foods are important to encourage and avoid is important. Another consideration is that after a stroke it can be difficult to eat because of the chaos of the hospital, difficulty swallowing and lack of energy and appetite, so some people become undernourished. Finally, if you cannot swallow, then your diet should be altered to help you to stay healthy and strong in the long run.

Diet and the prevention of stroke and heart disease

What do we know?

- Studies have shown that eating more fruit and vegetables decreases your risk for developing both heart disease and stroke. In areas of the UK where fruit and vegetables are eaten less, the incidence of stroke is much higher.
- Recent research suggests that it is the antioxidant properties of fruit and vegetables that help to prevent stroke and heart disease. Antioxidants help to prevent damage from oxidative free radicals – molecules that are thought to increase the formation of fatty plaques in the blood vessels. Antioxidants are thought to be beneficial even in diseases such as Parkinson's disease, Alzheimer's disease and chronic inflammatory disease.
- Salt is all too often poured plentifully onto food to make it taste better, but salt is directly linked to increased blood pressure. Salt does this by drawing water into the blood vessels,

making the volume of blood higher and therefore the blood pressure higher. It also encourages smooth muscle cells in the vessels to grow more, making the blood pressure higher.

- In addition, salt also makes the blood more likely to clot and increases the risk for stroke in this way.

Keeping strong after a stroke

It has been demonstrated that when you have a stroke there is a high chance that you will be undernourished even before the stroke, and that this state of poor nutrition gets worse after the stroke. Being undernourished means that the immune system (that is, the body's defence mechanism against infection) is lowered, and the likelihood of getting infections increases. In this vulnerable stage it is vital that nourishment be taken seriously before these complications have a chance to develop.

One of the great pleasures for many people is good food. After a stroke, the amount of tasty, good food eaten can become much less for a number of reasons.

- *Taste buds become less sensitive.* As a normal part of ageing, the senses of smell and taste become less sensitive, and so the vastly different tastes once enjoyed can become bland and uninteresting. This happens to different extents to different people as they become older.
- *Sweet things taste better.* Sensitivity to bitter and sweet extremes tend not to be affected, so many find themselves eating sweets and adding salt to their food to try to make the sensation of eating foods more appealing – both extremes of which are obviously bad in terms of increasing your risk for diabetes and high blood pressure. Be aware of why you might be eating unhealthy foods and try to avoid this as much as possible, within reason.
- *Neglected teeth.* Again, with old age, the state of dentition may worsen and dentures may need to be fitted. All too often, the

cleaning of teeth and the fitting of the right sized dentures is a problem, leading to what appears to be a lower appetite, when in reality it is just too arduous an experience to eat.

- *Poor swallowing.* If you are a family member, friend or carer, imagine how it must feel not to be able to savour the flavours of the food, but on top of this not to enjoy the textures of foods. Because the muscles that are responsible for swallowing foods may be affected in stroke, the person may have to have liquidized or semi-solid food until their muscles regain their strength. The sheer thought of more pureed food can lead to a person displaying a 'lack of appetite'. For someone who enjoys food – for that matter anyone who eats – going onto a soft diet can be very depressing and make one feel like a baby – helpless. There are ways of making the soft diet less depressing, however. If you are responsible for making the food, try it yourself! Make sure it tastes good. Try to show the person the meal before it is pureed, because this shows them what they are eating so that they can be conscious of the flavours and appreciate the tastes more.

- *Physical impairment.* Poor vision, poor spatial awareness, hand tremors and other effects of the stroke can make the physical act of picking up food or using cutlery difficult. If there is not enough time and there are not enough people to help you eat, then you end up eating less because you are dependent on someone else for food. In institutions such as care homes and hospitals, where time is short and meal times more controlled, poor nutrition may result.

- *Isolation.* On returning home you may suddenly feel very alone, after so much input from others at hospital. Many elderly and young people are lonely and isolated before their stroke, and this problem becomes worse after the stroke. The effects of social isolation, loneliness and depression can manifest as a poor appetite, and this should be taken very seriously to avoid malnourishment and the complications of poor nutrition.

- *Heavy smoking.* Smoking makes the taste buds less sensitive, so try to stop as early as possible if you want to enjoy the taste of food for longer!

What to eat

As you get older, your diet may become unhealthy unless you actively consider what you are eating and try to maintain a balanced healthy diet. It is even more important to be aware of what vitamins and minerals are in which foods, because these substances can improve your health and decrease risk factors in many ways. Here are some tips on where to get the right vitamins.

Vitamins C and E

These vitamins have excellent antioxidant properties. Most fruits contain vitamin C, famously oranges, but also blueberries, spinach, tomato, mango and many others. There are smaller amounts in liver and in milk. Vitamin E may be found in many vegetable and nut oils, as well as in peanuts, asparagus, tomatoes and many other fruits and vegetables.

Calcium and vitamin D

These are important to maintain bone strength and prevent osteoporosis, which causes weak bones. In the elderly, and especially after a stroke, the risk for falling and fracturing a bone is higher, and so having a good diet to make the bones stronger is important. Calcium is found in dairy products, seaweeds, nuts and seeds, beans, oranges, figs, soy milk and kale, as well as other sources. Vitamin D is found in fish oils and many fish, as well as in mushrooms and eggs.

Zinc

Zinc has been shown to be excellent for tissue healing, and is found in meat, beans, nuts, almonds, whole grains, pumpkin seeds and sunflower seeds.

Difficulty swallowing

Swallowing is a complex interaction between nerves and muscles, which co-ordinate the passage of food from the mouth to the back of the throat and down into the gut. In about 50 per cent of cases of stroke, there is some element of swallowing difficulty, ranging from complete inability to swallow to an impairment in swallowing. At first, instead of eating things through your mouth you may have to have fluids delivered through a drip or through a nasogastric (nose to stomach) tube.

The opening to the gut sits at the back of the throat right next to the opening to the airway. If there is impaired swallowing, then things in the mouth can slip into the airway rather than the gut, and the presence of these particles in the lungs can lead to infections. In a well person, sometimes the food particles pass into the airway but instantly you cough and splutter – this is a reflex that helps to prevent abnormal particles being lodged in the lung. However, this coughing or choking reflex does not always occur after a stroke, and so the particles go into the airways 'silently'. This is called 'aspiration', and can lead to a chest infection.

To assess your ability to swallow, the speech and language therapist will find out whether

- you choke or cough while eating;
- you have had chest infections;
- you have difficulty speaking; or
- you make unusual breathing noises while eating.

They will also take into account how conscious you are, how aware of your surroundings you are, how cooperative you are and how much the stroke has impaired your memory, language, speech and spatial awareness. Looking inside your mouth can reveal whether there are sores or other signs of inattention to the mouth.

Then they assess your swallowing, by giving you different consistencies of food, starting with solids, then pureed, then thickened liquids and then liquids. They assess the speed of eating, whether there is any choking or coughing, whether saliva is managed (i.e. whether there is drooling) and whether you are able to clear your throat and cough while eating. Another clue is the quality of the speech – if the voice sounds 'wet hoarse' after eating then this suggests incomplete swallowing.

The 'gold standard' test for assessing your swallowing is with videofluoroscopy, which is imaging while you swallow different consistencies, types, volumes, temperatures and tastes of foods, given by spoon or cup and at different speeds. It shows the extent of dysfunction of the swallowing, and guides the speech and language therapist to make a care plan for eating. If there is a milder difficulty, then liquids may be thickened. If there is a severe difficulty, then it may be appropriate to place a nasogastric tube until your swallowing technique has improved. In very severe cases, a gastrostomy tube is placed, which is a tube from the outside of the stomach, directly through the abdomen and into the stomach. This can be used short term or, if swallowing does not improve, long term.

Top tips for ... helping with swallowing

- Ensure that the bed head is elevated and at 90 degrees while you are eating.
- Have supervised meals.
- Try to cough and clear your throat while you are eating and even when you are not eating to improve the strength of the muscles.
- Try to make sure that the rate of delivery of food is not too fast.
- Do exercises by moving your mouth, tongue and lips to improve the strength of your muscles.
- Sometimes medication can be given to prevent saliva drooling; ask your doctor about this.

9

Psychology and stroke

It's OK to feel sad

Understandably, a certain amount of sadness is to be expected after a stroke. It is important that you allow yourself to grieve. It is perfectly reasonable to feel sad about impairment or loss of abilities. Allow yourself to express your sadness, by talking to loved ones or talking to a counsellor. Obviously, when distress or grief are prolonged, they may become manifestations of clinical depression. In the aftermath of a stroke, try to speak to others, address negative feelings and use the positive techniques mentioned below to help work through these feelings.

Try to take up the activities that you used to enjoy. Even if you cannot do the knitting or the singing that you used to do, there may still be ways to enjoy them. Spending time with the people with whom you used to share activities, taking part as much as possible, watching others or reading or learning about your interest – these are all basic ways to maintain your interest. If the interest cannot be taken up again, then try to think of things that you were interested in doing in the past, which you now may be able to do – perhaps you have more time to read or write, so why not have a go? People take up all sorts of activities, from painting to poetry, after a stroke.

Some people find that writing their feelings down helps them to cope with difficult emotions. Recording thoughts on a tape or asking someone to listen to them can be useful. Reading self-help books or doing online cognitive behavioural therapy – a form of counselling – may improve your psychological state.

Building supportive relationships is necessary to get through the rehabilitation process. Whether you like it or not, you need to be aware of your own vulnerability as an individual. Relationships with others help you to reflect on your own situation and bounce your thoughts off them. Being a support to someone else who is in need can improve your own feeling of self worth, so be there for your friends and family as you used to. Information and feedback help people to understand themselves better, and expressing emotions helps to manage stress. Some people need social interaction more than others; some need close relationships more than others. After a stroke it can feel as if the existing social support is lacking, or it may even be too much. However, remember that – apart from the family you have and the health professionals around you – there are a wealth of people in the community, in the outside world, to meet and several social activities if you look out for them.

Family members and carers can feel as if they are dealing with a different person after a stroke. People react in different ways to the stress of a stroke, and the commonest feelings are those of sadness and frustration. In order to deal with these feelings, sometimes a person can appear to be behaving differently from his or her usual personality. For example, some people become over-optimistic and try too hard to do things that they cannot do, pushing themselves too far and ending up putting themselves at risk by doing so. Others are pessimistic about the future, and become de-motivated and quiet. Neither approach is an ideal way to deal with the aftermath of a stroke, but they are both only natural. Imagine the person who was a plumber, an artist or a doctor who is now unable to use the most important tools of his or her trade – the hands, eyes or voice. This can be devastating, and so it is vital that family members and carers be sympathetic, and bear the person's background in mind in order to understand what he or she has lost.

Common feelings after a stroke are as follows:

- frustration
- anxiety

- anger
- apathy
- depression.

There is evidence that major life changes convey high stress-related health risk for a period of two to eighteen months after the event. Stress-related illnesses such as depression and anxiety are therefore more common. Your doctor may ask you a series of screening questions to find out whether your feelings are indicative of depression. If depression is the cause for your change in personality, then it may be that you need counselling or medical treatment.

Depression

Lying in bed, feeling helpless and unable to do the things that you used to be able to do, while being dependent on people who may be younger than you, perhaps family members that once were looked after by you, can lead to feelings of sadness and guilt. This is to be expected after going through such a traumatic experience. However, if these feelings persist then they may indicate that you are becoming clinically depressed. Studies have shown that there is a risk for depression after stroke, but often this is not diagnosed because the symptoms of the stroke take over the management plan, and your feelings are not fully assessed. Diagnosing depression and treating it can improve your quality of life after a stroke and improve your rehabilitation potential. This is because two of the symptoms of depression are low motivation and low insight, and it can make you feel very tired. All of these factors will hinder rehabilitation.

However, although it is to be expected that you will feel sad after having a stroke, this does not mean that you have depression. Depression means that these symptoms last for weeks or even months. You may feel low all of the time and no longer be able to find any pleasure in the activities that you once enjoyed.

The following are other symptoms of depression that you should be aware of:

- reduced energy
- feeling tired all of the time
- little interest in pleasures previously enjoyed
- poor sleep and early waking
- decreased appetite and weight loss
- lost interest in sex
- difficulty concentrating
- feeling worried and restless
- feeling tense and anxious
- feeling less confident
- avoiding other people
- feeling worthless
- feeling hopeless
- feeling guilty
- thinking about suicide.

If these feelings occur for weeks, then they are very serious, and if a person is thinking about suicide then this must be assessed in greater detail. There is no harm in talking to someone about their thoughts about suicide. People are afraid to ask these questions, but talking about it does not increase the chances of it happening; instead it helps the person to talk through their feelings.

Treatment for depression begins with the doctor assessing how severe the symptoms are. Sometimes a person has mild symptoms and can make changes to his or her lifestyle to improve this, for example taking up exercise or a social activity. Talking about any concerns can help to open up feelings that are difficult to express and allow the person to discuss ways to resolve their feelings by themselves. There are also self-help groups that provide support through social activities. The Stroke Association and other charities have information on local support groups, and it is often helpful to chat with other people with the same condition. There are also self-help books and websites that some people find useful. (See Useful contacts at the end of this book.)

In some cases, the doctor will suggest a course of antidepressants. There is, for many people, a considerable stigma attached to taking medication or with being diagnosed as having depression, but depression is a very common and treatable illness, and it is not worth holding back from adequate treatment because of this stigma. Many people stay on antidepressants for a short time and are then able to live their lives symptom free. Antidepressants take two to four weeks to take effect. If the first antidepressant does not work, then the dose may be changed or a different medication tried instead. Antidepressants are not addictive but withdrawal symptoms are quite common if you stop taking them suddenly or if you miss a dose.

Some people do not need antidepressants – a short course of counselling may be enough. There are more complex forms of therapy, such as CBT (cognitive behavioural therapy), which allows the person to talk through his or her feelings and recognize why they feel a certain way, and then work out ways to change negative emotions. CBT is based on the principle that the way we feel is partly dependent on the way we think about things, and it suggests ways of thinking and behaving that challenge negative thoughts.

In very severe depression, some people will be referred to a specialist psychiatrist or a community mental health team to assess fully their needs and see whether more specialist or intensive therapy is needed. The team includes psychologists, doctors, nurses and social workers.

Anxiety

Depression and anxiety are closely related illnesses that may occur at the same time. People with anxiety disorder are physically and emotionally affected by anxiety over matters about which other people would not normally become anxious.

If you are walking home from work and feel that someone dangerous is following you, you become concerned, your heart rate starts to increase and you walk faster, with your senses more alert to danger. As the person approaches these physical changes increase, so that your heart is racing, you sweat and breathe faster, thinking about what may happen next. The same sorts of feelings are triggered in anxiety disorder, but they occur often, even without a trigger, or with minor incidents. Panic attacks are another expression of anxiety disorder.

Symptoms of anxiety

The symptoms of anxiety include the following:

- palpitations
- sweating
- trembling/shaking
- sensation of choking or shortness of breath
- chest pain or discomfort
- feeling sick
- abdominal pain
- dizziness
- feeling of things being unreal or of the person being unreal
- fear of going crazy or losing control
- fear of dying
- numb feelings or tingling sensation
- chills and hot flushes.

It is a combination of these symptoms that persist for a long time with no medical cause behind them that leads to a diagnosis of anxiety. The same physical symptoms of changed sleep pattern and change in appetite that occur in depression occur in anxiety.

Treating anxiety

Anxiety can be managed by breathing exercises, also known as diaphragmatic breathing. Slow deep breathing lowers the heart rate and, if used often, can be a very useful long-term therapy.

Taking up exercise can also help to relieve stress and anxiety, and so can having a good laugh (known as humour skills). Different things make people laugh, but making an effort to find out what things make someone happy and make them laugh might help them to manage their sad feelings or worries after a stroke. Positive respites can help – going somewhere peaceful or spending quality time with someone. Again, this is absurdly simple, but if it works when a person is well then why would it not work when he or she is ill? In some cases, anxiety can be treated with medications as well as counselling.

Personality changes

Someone who has had a stroke can often seem as though he or she has had a change in personality, and can sometimes appear to act irrationally, perhaps showing unwarranted anger or resentment towards family and friends. Often this is as a result of the brain injury, but may be worsened by the person's situation. Upsetting as it may be, if you are caring for someone who's had a stroke, try not to take it personally. It is important to remember that a person will 'return to their old self' as their rehabilitation progresses. Be prepared for changed behaviour. Sometimes people who have had a stroke respond to their anger and sad feelings by becoming violent or behaving inappropriately in other ways. This can be very distressing for the people who know them well. If it becomes to difficult to cope with, friends and family members should remember that your social worker and doctor are there to discuss problems, and care packages can be altered accordingly.

Mood swings

After a stroke it can be quite common for emotions to go from one extreme to the other, for example from being tearful to being suddenly angry. Part of this might be because of the stress and anxiety experienced after a stroke, while still trying to keep hold of all of the things that are important to you – relationships with people, your job and more. However, mood swings are quite often due to the brain injury itself and can therefore be difficult to control. An appreciation that mood changes occur as a result of the stroke may make it easier for people around you to understand, and so avoid embarrassment and upset. There are no hard and fast rules, but what you can do is make family members aware that mood swings can be really difficult to cope with, and they often take up a lot of energy and time for the person who has had a stroke as well as their family. Those who are caring for someone after a stroke should be sympathetic and reassure the person and remind him or her that their emotions are swinging because of the stroke.

Fatigue

After a stroke you might feel tired all the time and find that small tasks suddenly take a lot more effort. It is normal to feel tired after a long period of being immobile, or hardly moving at all, but it is important not to become overtired in an effort to try to get back to usual. After a tiring task, you should always take time to rest. Taking regular breaks will also help to conserve your energy.

Look at other reasons for being tired. Is it poor sleep or caused by medications? Tiredness is also a symptom of anxiety and depression. Look at the list of symptoms in the earlier sections on these conditions. If any of those symptoms are occurring, then consultation with a doctor is important to rule them out.

Make sure that you are getting adequate nutrition. A poor diet will lead to lower energy levels. There are also relaxation techniques that you can use to overcome fatigue, such as meditation, or complementary remedies such as aromatherapy.

10

Preventing further strokes: causes and risks

There are many reasons to change your life after a stroke. Many people recover their usual activities after rehabilitation and take the experience of the stroke as a 'wake-up call' to reassess their life and prioritize their health and happiness, doing activities that they always wished to do and enjoying life more. This is a great attitude to have and is doubly important because improving your lifestyle can dramatically decrease your chances of having a further stroke. For example, a person who has had a mini-stroke – a TIA (transient ischaemic attack) – is ten times more likely to have a stroke than a person who has never had a TIA, regardless of age. Whatever your age, though, it is never too late to change your lifestyle.

Modern medicine is governed by research, which – among other things – can generate enough clinical evidence to say whether something is responsible for a disease or not, or whether a treatment is effective. This means that only when a treatment has been proven to work does it start to be used to treat a disease. There have been many medicines that have been found to reduce the risk for a person developing a stroke. More important than evidence about medications, however, is that preventing the disease by modifying lifestyle and reducing risk factors has been proven to be possible. Now doctors spend a substantial proportion of their consultation time advising people on how to reduce their risk. Consider the following definitions.

- *Primary prevention* = preventing a disease developing by controlling blood pressure, blood sugar and so on.

- *Secondary prevention* = having had a stroke, starting aspirin and other tablets to prevent recurrence.
- *Tertiary prevention* = having had a stroke, undergoing surgery to clear the carotid artery.

As you can see from these brief descriptions, the more time invested in primary care, the less are the chances of having to receive more life-impinging treatments.

The risk for vascular disease (such as stroke and heart attacks) is increased 70 to 200 per cent in people who smoke one pack of cigarettes per day. Therefore, it makes sense to stop smoking or at least cut down. If you read about heart attacks, the same risk factors such as smoking will be described, and so controlling the risk factors for stroke means you are also reducing your risk for all other vascular diseases. By improving your lifestyle you will reduce your overall risk for what we term 'cerebrovascular' (the brain and the vessels), 'cardiovascular' (the heart and the vessels) and peripheral vascular (the small vessels in the limbs) diseases.

As the name suggests, modifiable risk factors means you can change them to decrease the likelihood of having another stroke or heart attack. Obviously, for people with many years of habit and routine, it can be a real challenge to change their lifestyle. It can seem as if all the nice things in life must be stopped – comfortable habits such as smoking, a fatty diet and a sedentary lifestyle. Also, the older people get, the more set in their ways they tend to be.

So how do you turn your life upside down? Well, a stroke itself is often the impetus for change, but why not change your life before a stroke happens, once you have counted the number of risk factors on one or two hands? Replace the terms 'smoking', 'fatty diet' and 'sedentary lifestyle' with 'fresh air', 'regular exercise' and 'delicious healthy diet' – don't they sound much better?

In this chapter we will go through ways in which you can change your lifestyle, but it is no good reading without wanting to change. It is very easy for doctors to drone on and on about healthy lifestyles, but it won't make a dot of difference if the person being addressed doesn't have the motivation to change. So if that's you, then you need to adopt a change-embracing attitude before reading on. If you can't adopt such an attitude, then I hope at least that some of the examples below will help you to make the decision to change, and make steps toward change – even if it's only a tiny change. Every little change makes a difference, and nothing will happen overnight. It takes time to change your lifestyle, so persevere and expect failure a few times before achieving your health goals.

What risk factors for stroke cannot be changed?

Unfortunately, some people are at risk without any obvious risk factors. That is because research has shown that certain factors that are totally out of a person's control put them at greater risk for having a stroke.

- As a person gets older, he or she is more likely to have a stroke. The risk for having a stroke approximately doubles for each decade of life after age 55 years.
- Certain ethnicities have a higher incidence of stroke, for example people of African, Caribbean or Asian descent have a higher risk for stroke than do Caucasian people. This is related to the higher incidence of high blood pressure and diabetes in these ethnic groups.
- If you have a family member who has had a stroke, then there is an increased risk that you will have a stroke. This could be because of a genetic predisposition to vascular disease.
- Men are more likely to have a stroke than women.
- Women who use birth control pills and who are pregnant have a very slightly increased risk for stroke.

- Already having some form of heart disease or a previous stroke is a risk factor for a further stroke.

Modifiable risk factors

Many risk factors for stroke can be reduced or stopped completely. These are known as modifiable risk factors and include the following:

- high blood pressure
- smoking
- diabetes
- high cholesterol
- obesity
- atrial fibrillation
- alcohol
- carotid artery disease.

High blood pressure

High blood pressure, also known as hypertension, is a very important risk factor for stroke. Since the introduction of drugs to control blood pressure, the number of deaths caused by strokes has declined, and many people think that the better control of the nation's blood pressure is one of the key reasons for this change.

Why do people get high blood pressure?

Most people have what is known as 'essential hypertension', which is high blood pressure with no known cause. Some people are more likely to have essential hypertension because they have a family history of it, and there is some evidence that genetic factors can increase the likelihood that hypertension will develop. As well as this, being overweight, smoking, having diabetes, high alcohol intake, kidney disease, excessive salt intake, lack of exercise and certain medicines can all contribute to rising blood pressure.

Ten per cent of people have an underlying cause for their high blood pressure, and this is called 'secondary hypertension'. The main causes are kidney disease, alcohol abuse and hormone problems.

What is blood pressure?

Blood pressure is a measure of how much pressure the blood vessels are under. There are two numbers. The top number is the higher number because this is the pressure in the vessels when the heart is pumping out blood. The second number is lower because this is the pressure when the heart is relaxing, and the vessels are under much less pressure. High blood pressure is diagnosed once three separate measurements, taken on different occasions, show that blood pressure is above 140/90. The higher the blood pressure and the longer the period of time that a person has high blood pressure, the higher is the risk for stroke. If you have diabetes, then you should be aiming for an even lower blood pressure of 130/80, because the combination of diabetes and high blood pressure increases your risk for stroke further.

Many people associate the words high blood pressure with being stressed, and although it is not a well researched factor, it is known that if someone is under stress or strain then their blood pressure will temporarily increase. This is an adrenaline response, which is a natural way for the body to cope with stress. Although the evidence for a link between stress and blood pressure is poor, there is no harm in trying to make your life less stressful – even if it doesn't lower your blood pressure, why not change your lifestyle to make it more manageable and make yourself happier?

How is blood pressure related to stroke?

High blood pressure slowly damages the blood vessels. The mechanism by which this happens is unclear but what we do know is that the long-term effect of chronically high blood pressure is hardening of the blood vessel walls and damage to small vessels. A good example of this is to look at the back of the eyes of a person who has high blood pressure. When you look into the eye of someone who has had high blood pressure for years with an ophthalmoscope (an instrument used to look at the retina at the back of the eye), you can see blood vessels with thickened walls, a more twisted appearance and cholesterol deposits in the vessels, which lead to smaller vessel diameters and hardened thickened vessel walls. Little spots where bleeds have occurred and where the blood supply has been blocked off because of damage to the vessels can also be seen. Imagine this on a larger scale throughout the body, and the brain. This long-term damage to the vessels leads to ischaemia (lack of blood supply to tissues), which can result in a heart attack or stroke. Sometimes, the chronic high blood pressure leads to outpouchings of blood vessels in the brain, which burst under the pressure, and this leads to haemorrhagic stroke.

Treatment of high blood pressure

Many things influence how high a person's blood pressure is. The relationship between heart disease, smoking, cholesterol, diabetes and obesity is complex, and the likelihood is that if you have any of those risk factors your blood pressure may be higher. This is because smoking and diabetes cause damage to the small vessels, thus increasing the blood pressure. Obesity may mean that you do less exercise and are at higher risk for high blood pressure. Heart disease puts a strain on the heart, which then has to work harder – this may also lead to increased blood pressure.

This is why when you see your doctor to have your blood pressure checked, one of the first 'treatments' is lifestyle advice.

Simple changes in lifestyle can reduce your blood pressure without you having to use medication. Also, stopping smoking will lower your blood pressure (that's one risk factor sorted) as well as remove another major risk factor from your list (that's two!). Ways to reduce blood pressure include the following:

- healthy eating
- low sodium/salt diet
- lose weight
- take up exercise
- stop smoking
- try to reduce stress
- reduce your alcohol intake.

However, if your blood pressure remains high despite these measures, then blood pressure tablets may be prescribed. Depending on your age, ethnicity and other medical problems, different tablets may be given. Sometimes one tablet does not work alone, and so another one is given at the same time. Because the medications may have side effects, blood tests may be necessary before and during the administration of these medications. Here is a brief summary of the antihypertensive (blood pressure lowering) medications you might receive.

- *Diuretics*. These lower your blood pressure by affecting your salt-water balance and make you urinate more to get rid of water in the body.
- *Beta-blockers*. These drugs act on receptors in the heart and in the blood vessels, which make the heart beat slower and the blood vessels more relaxed, lowering the pressure in vessels.
- *ACE (angiotensin-converting enzyme) inhibitors and angiotensin antagonists*. ACE inhibitors act on the kidney and make the blood vessels relax, lowering the blood pressure overall.
- *Calcium channel blockers*. These block calcium channels, which usually make the heart and blood vessels constrict. Blocking these channels makes the blood vessels and heart relax.

- *Vasodilators*. Vasodilators act on the muscle in blood vessel walls, making the blood vessels enlarge, thus reducing the pressure of the blood carried in the vessels.

There are other more rarely used medications used to lower blood pressure. Remember that once you start these medications, it is not impossible to lower your blood pressure using lifestyle changes, so keep trying. Occasionally, your doctor may stop blood pressure medications if you have succeeded in lowering your blood pressure yourself, for example by maintaining a healthy diet. Make sure that you get your blood pressure rechecked if you change your lifestyle. Regular blood pressure checks are necessary to make sure your blood pressure is not getting *too* low or even higher, requiring adjustments to be made to the dose of medications.

Smoking

Campaigns to improve awareness of the health conditions caused by smoking have helped people to understand that smoking is linked to heart disease and lung cancer. This is just a fraction of the diseases caused by smoking. Stroke is another to add to the list of reasons why, if you are a smoker, stopping smoking should be a priority.

How smoking causes strokes

Cigarettes contribute to the formation of fatty plaques in the arteries. Smoking doubles the risk for ischaemic stroke. Even without any other risk factor, by smoking alone your risk is more than double that of someone who does not smoke. The way cigarettes do this is by

- making the vessels less compliant and distensible
- increasing blood levels of fibrinogen, which encourages clot formation
- increasing blood haematocrit, which increases the risk for clot formation

- increasing platelet aggregation (platelets help form clots)
- lowering the levels of high-density lipoprotein, which – if high – is protective against stroke.

It is a vicious cycle of risk factors. Smoking causes high blood pressure. Both smoking and high blood pressure lead to fatty deposits in the vessels. The delicate inside lining of the blood vessels is slowly damaged by the cigarette smoke. This makes the lining 'rougher', so that it is easier for fats to catch on the rough inside lining of the vessels and build up slowly over time. Eventually, the walls of the arteries become covered in a fatty mass called an 'atheroma', also known as a clot. If the clot dislodges, then it may be carried by the bloodstream into the brain or the heart, and cause heart attacks or strokes.

Smoking is also linked to higher cholesterol levels and high blood pressure. So, by stopping smoking, other risk factors are better controlled simultaneously.

In a study that looked at the arteries of people aged 15 to 34 who had died in accidents, suicides or murders, those who had smoked had much more fatty change in their arteries compared with those who had not smoked. There were more arteries covered in small plaques of fat, which is surprising considering their relatively young age. In some smokers' arteries, fat was squeezed out of the arteries 'like paste'. What this means is that, from a young age, smoking makes you more likely to build up fatty plaques in your arteries. This is one example of a study that has related smoking to vascular disease, and there are hundreds more. Modern medicine is built on evidence – if we have enough evidence that there is a causative effect, then we can start telling people to cut down the thing that we *know* is making their illness worse, and smoking ticks all the wrong boxes.

Smoking and chronic lung disease

When you smoke, you may have a smoker's cough. This is because smoking causes irritation in the delicate linings of the airways. In the long term the effect of continued smoking can cause chronic lung disease – diseases that used to be known as emphysema and bronchitis. The inflammation in the lungs makes the airways stiff, so that breathing in is harder and then breathing out waste gases is harder still; therefore, there is never enough oxygen in the lungs getting into the body. This chronic low level of oxygen in the blood makes the heart have to work harder to get oxygen to all of the tissues, and it is therefore more likely that you will have a heart attack or a stroke. Cigarettes contain carbon monoxide, which – when inhaled – also reduces the amount of oxygen in the bloodstream, making the heart work harder still and putting the blood vessels under more pressure to compensate for the low oxygen levels.

That is why you see many people with lung disease secondary to smoking getting short of breath on mild exertion, and in some cases having to use oxygen all of the time.

Environmental smoke

Nearly 90 per cent of *non-smokers* who have a stroke have detectable nicotine in their blood, caused by environmental smoke. So, if you live with a smoker, then make it a priority to help them to quit with you, or at least encourage the smoker to smoke outside. You can tell them that the risk for having a heart attack decreases by 50 per cent after one year of stopping smoking. After five years the risk is the same as that in someone who has never smoked. *So it is never too late!*

Giving up smoking

The relaxing effects of smoking a cigarette are caused by the fact that nicotine is a stimulant, which you get used to having. When deprived of that relaxed feeling, you get withdrawal symptoms.

Your heart races and you feel sweaty and anxious. Taking a cigarette stops these withdrawal symptoms temporarily. It is worth understanding that this is why quitting is so hard – because you feel you need a cigarette all the time. This also means that when you decide to cut down, these feelings will persist, worsen and make it doubly hard not to go back to smoking.

Before you decide to stop smoking, you really have to want to stop smoking, and to understand that you will feel bad while you are cutting down. There is no need to feel like a failure when you do go back to smoking because many people attempt to quit multiple times before they actually succeed, and the effort counts for a lot. Keep trying when you fail.

Top tips for ... giving up smoking

- Decide to stop smoking yourself. It's no good being nagged by someone else if you are not interested yourself in stopping.
- Take things one day at a time.
- Don't be disheartened if you quit and then start smoking again. Just try quitting again and again.
- Tell your family and friends that you are quitting, and ask them kindly not to smoke around you!
- Remove all of your smoking apparatus and any reminders of your old habit that might be in your house.
- Make a note of how much money you save at the end of each week from not smoking, and get yourself a treat when you reach a certain amount of potential money not spent on cigarettes.
- Use chewing gum or a sweet if you feel the need to put something in your mouth.
- Give yourself a pat on the back at the end of each day without smoking.
- Try to manage situations where you may feel pressure to smoke socially, for example parties or other social gatherings.
- Quit smoking with a friend to encourage each other.
- Take up a sport or hobby to help preoccupy your time while you quit smoking.

Once you do stop smoking, you'll inevitably start getting a nasty cough – this is a normal part of withdrawal. Eventually, over time, your breathing will feel much easier, and exercise will not make you as short of breath as it might have done before. This is because smoking irritates the lining of the lungs, causing them to secrete inflammatory substances that tickle the airways and clog them up, and it takes a long time (sometimes up to a year) for this reaction to subside.

Other benefits include increased energy and better appreciation of food, because smoking makes your taste buds insensitive to flavours.

Finally there is a great sense of achievement. Your family and friends will no longer be at risk because of your smoking, and neither will you.

Other ways to stop smoking may be advised by your doctor. For example, the NHS (National Health Service) provides Stop Smoking groups, where you meet others who are quitting, do exercises to help quit smoking and receive counselling. Some people use nicotine replacement skin patches or chewing gum to help them to quit smoking initially. These can be weaned off slowly to help prevent the symptoms of withdrawal while quitting smoking. Some people respond well to alternative therapies such as hypnotherapy or acupuncture.

Diabetes mellitus

Diabetes is essentially high blood sugar. Non-insulin-dependent diabetes mellitus (type 2 diabetes) is the most common type of diabetes in the Western world. Type 2 diabetes reduces your body's ability to control blood sugar. It is a major cause of early death, heart disease, kidney disease, stroke and blindness. People with diabetes have a higher risk for having other risk factors, such as high blood pressure, obesity and high cholesterol. Controlling blood sugar also prevents complications of diabetes such as eye disease, kidney disease, peripheral vascular disease and foot sores.

This condition can also increase the risk for stroke as a result of damage to the blood vessels after longstanding high blood sugar. The high blood sugar slowly damages the small vessels.

Many people with diabetes also have high blood pressure and high blood cholesterol, and are overweight. This means that their risk is increased more. Better control of the other risk factors as well as maintaining a low blood sugar in diabetes decreases the chances of long-term damage to the vessels.

High cholesterol

What is cholesterol?

Cholesterol is part of the diet and is used by the body in various ways, including manufacture of natural hormones and for vitamin D. Most of our cholesterol is produced by the liver and transported to other tissues, but on top of this we often ingest too much cholesterol, and when there is too much cholesterol in the body it ends up depositing itself on the walls of blood vessels.

Types of cholesterol

There are three types of cholesterol. High-density lipoprotein (HDL) is actually protective against stroke. LDL (low-density lipoprotein) and triglycerides increase the risk for stroke. Current guidelines in the UK recommend a total cholesterol level under 5 mmol/l, and an LDL level under 3 mmol/l.

How cholesterol is related to stroke

Where the blood vessel walls are damaged as a result of diabetes, high blood pressure or smoking, the cholesterol easily fastens itself to the rough inside walls of the vessels. This causes fatty plaques to develop on the vessel walls – a process called 'atherosclerosis'. The fatty plaques become clot, which can break off and deposit anywhere in the body, causing strokes, heart attacks and other vascular disease.

As the cholesterol builds up, the vessels become narrower. Fat builds up on the vessel walls, especially when the cholesterol level in the blood is high. Imagine a tube under pressure. If you make the tube narrower the pressure in the tube gets higher, and so higher cholesterol contributes to high blood pressure.

If the blood vessels become narrowed because of cholesterol, this causes lack of oxygen to the tissues and the death of the tissues, causing a stroke or heart attack.

What causes high blood cholesterol?

- As well as dietary intake of cholesterol-rich foods, the other cause of high cholesterol is smoking, which has been shown to increase the levels of LDL cholesterol.
- Some people have medical disorders that increase their cholesterol levels, such as hypothyroidism, genetically inherited familial hypercholesterolaemia and disorders of the clotting system.
- Excess alcohol is also known to increase levels of cholesterol. People who are overweight are also more likely to have high cholesterol.

Medications for high cholesterol

As with other prevention strategies, the first step to lower cholesterol is to try the lifestyle changes mentioned earlier, but if this doesn't work then sometimes medication can be given to lower cholesterol levels. Doctors use a risk assessment score that takes into account all of your risk factors to determine how important it is for you to take a statin, which lowers cholesterol. However, if your cholesterol level is high then cholesterol-lowering tablets may be required in any case. The main side effect of these tablets is that they can rarely cause muscle pains due to inflammation of the muscles.

Obesity

Being overweight is related to stroke because there is a higher incidence of diabetes, high blood pressure, high cholesterol and low exercise levels, as well as poor diet. When someone has a BMI (body mass index) greater than 30, they are obese, and the risk for many diseases is greatly increased.

To find out whether someone is obese, a measure of the height and the weight is needed to calculate the BMI. The BMI is the weight (in kilograms) divided by the height (in metres) squared.

- BMI under 18.5 = underweight
- BMI of 18.5 to 24.9 = normal weight
- BMI of 25 to 29.9 = overweight
- BMI of 30 or greater = obesity.

If you are in the higher categories, then reducing your weight by just ten per cent can have a dramatic influence on your other risk factors.

Sarah

Sarah had a BMI of 32 and went to see her doctor to talk about her weight. A routine blood pressure check revealed that she had high blood pressure, of 160/80. Her doctor explained the risks of having a high blood pressure and advised her that if she lost some weight this could also help to lower her blood pressure. He went through her diet and advised her to stop frying foods, stop eating 'junk food' and takeaways, and instead of having a full English breakfast to eat fruit for breakfast, as a start.

Sarah found it very difficult to change her diet, and on her next trip to the doctor was disappointed to find she had not lost weight and her blood pressure was the same. The doctor advised her that to avoid having to take medication to lower her blood pressure she should have another go at sticking to the dietary advice. He also provided her with a discount gym pass, which is available to people who have a need for exercise on medical grounds.

Sarah went to the gym regularly and took on board the dietary advice, and managed to lose five kilograms. On the next visit to the doctor her blood pressure was 145/80. She was advised to keep up her current activities and work toward a gradual weight loss to avoid redeveloping her high blood pressure, and try to reduce her BMI further.

Modifying your diet

Changing the usual shopping list is much harder than it looks at first. Have a look at your usual shopping list, and then go through each food and see if you could change it for a healthier option. For example, instead of buying full-fat milk, you can change to half-fat milk. Eating the wrong foods is easy to do, and after years of buying the same foods and cooking them the same way, it is frustrating to have to learn a new way of eating. For many people, however, this provides an opportunity to try new foods and to experiment with different ways of cooking delicious food from scratch. In addition, one of the bonuses of changing diet if you share food with a family, flatmates or friends is that you can work together to change your collective diets and make a difference to the health of a greater number of people instead of you alone. Consider the following items as things that need to change.

Fatty foods

There are two types of fat – saturated and unsaturated. You should avoid food that contains saturated fats, because these fats directly increase the level of LDL cholesterol in your blood.

There is absolutely no cholesterol in fruit and vegetables, and so replacing breakfast or desserts with fruit is a fantastic idea, and incorporating more vegetables in place of fatty cuts of meat in your dinner will make you feel satisfied and healthy simultaneously.

Foods that are high in unsaturated fats can help to improve your cholesterol, in moderation. Omega-3 fatty acids are known to increase the levels of 'good' (HDL) cholesterol in the blood. So eating more oily fish as part of your diet is an excellent move. To increase the levels of good cholesterol in your blood you should eat more of the following:

- oily fish
- avocados
- nuts and seeds
- sunflower, rapeseed and olive oil.

Check the labels of foods to see whether they are high in unsaturated fats rather than saturated fats.

Fibre

The level of HDL ('good cholesterol') in your blood is increased by eating high fibre foods such as

- cereal
- bread
- whole grain pasta
- brown rice.

Fruit and vegetables

As well as containing zero cholesterol, fruit and vegetables contain minerals as well as antioxidant vitamins such as E and C, which prevent oxidative damage to vessel walls.

Dieting

Crash diets (cutting out several foods at one time) do not work. It is better to make a dietary plan that includes a balance of fruit, vegetables, meat, fish and carbohydrates, and stick to it. Although dairy products and meat have their bad points, it is not necessary to totally cut these foods out. Just have them occasionally rather than every day. In most cases crash diets result in failure because it is much too difficult to change your diet so dramatically and so quickly.

If you are changing your diet, then make sure that the people who live with you, your family and friends, and your work colleagues know that you are trying to be more healthy, so that you can work together and they can encourage you to maintain the healthy diet you are aiming toward.

Many people are spurred on to reduce their cholesterol level without using medication, and it isn't that difficult to do. People go from a high to a normal cholesterol level just by taking regular exercise and switching to a healthier diet. Losing weight, giving up smoking and decreasing alcohol intake can dramatically alter your LDL and triglyceride levels.

Salt

The maximum salt intake each day should be about one teaspoon, or 0.2 oz. However, salt is included in many prepackaged and processed foods, and it is impossible to say how much salt is added to takeaway or restaurant foods, but everyone knows that adding salt to a bland food makes it tastier, so it is safer to be wary of any food that you haven't cooked yourself. Try to avoid putting salt on food and instead use other flavours, spices and herbs to make food tastier.

Your new shopping list

Some example shopping lists, highlighting items that tend to raise bad (LDL) cholesterol alongside alternatives that can lower it, are presented in Table 2 on the next page.

Exercise

Trying to lose weight by exercising alone or dieting alone seldom works. The best option is to try to consolidate the effects of a healthy diet with regular exercise.

Table 2 Your new shopping list

Your old shopping list (raising your bad cholesterol)	Your new shopping list (lowering your bad cholesterol)
Oil for frying food	Less oil: try grilling, baking, boiling or steaming food
Eggs for breakfast	Fibre (e.g. bananas, brown rice, wheat/bran and other cereals topped with fresh fruit)
Fatty meats	Oily fish
Full-fat milk	Skimmed milk
Margarines that contain saturated fat	Cholesterol-lowering butters
Crate of beer	Glass of wine
Cakes, biscuits and chocolate	More fresh fruit and vegetables
Salt	Lower your salt by using herbs and spices instead
Vegetable fats	Oils with several polyunsaturated fats; for instance, sunflower and nut oils will raise levels of HDL cholesterol
Fried foods and takeaways	Freshly cooked foods
Pastries and pies	Nuts and seeds
Sugar	Sweetener

Exercise gets your heart muscles and blood vessels used to higher levels of strain on the heart. The heart gets pumping, the blood vessels become stretched, and over time the heart and vessels adapt to the increased level of activity to work better under strain as well as at rest. If you check the heart rate of an athlete, it is much lower than that in the average person, because the heart is so healthy that it can beat at a lower rate to maintain a healthy blood pressure and maintain a good level of oxygen supply to the tissues.

The type of exercise you do doesn't matter, but try to do half an hour of exercise per day at least, and make it an exercise that makes you sweat at least a little. It can be any activity from walking to dancing to group sport.

After a stroke it is important to consider what exercise you can do and to discuss this with your occupational therapist or doctor. Overstretching yourself is dangerous. If you go to a gym, for example, explain to the gym instructor that you have had a stroke and what limbs were or still are affected, so that the exercises can be tailored accordingly.

Increased physical activity is associated with a lower risk for having a stroke. The problem is that as you get older, the energy required to do an activity increases. This can make it all too easy to become lazy and to ask someone else to do tasks for you. Then, after a stroke has happened, the setbacks are worse still – if someone else does everything for you, then you could get into the habit of depending on them, and even when you are fully recovered you may expect things to be done for you. In a study of 60- to 69-year-olds, 70 per cent of them reported that they took part in no physical outdoor activity at all, and this number increased in the older age groups. I met an elderly man who lived alone but had carers coming in every day after he had had a stroke, and he told me that his only activity was to watch TV and to buy from the TV buying channel, despite being able to walk with a stick after his stroke. I was surprised, because he had a positive attitude overall, but the reality was that – on further questioning – he had no one to come and take him out; his family members had all passed away, and he was frightened of his neighbours. So the reasons for decreased physical activity are often very complex and quite sad. For those lucky enough to have a supportive group of people around them, this situation can be avoided. For those who do not there are many support groups, as well as voluntary organizations and social services, that can help get you back outside. (See Useful contacts, at the end of this book.)

Top tips for ... getting some exercise

- Do it daily – make it your priority to do 30 minutes of exercise per day.
- You don't have to do strenuous exercise. Try walking or just lifting your legs while sitting in a chair.
- Spend less time on activities that use little energy, like watching television.
- Break your exercise up. If you get tired after 5 minutes, then do small bursts of exercise every so often during the day.
- Get an exercise partner so that you can encourage each other to exercise.
- Join an exercise class.
- If you can't stand physical exercise, then take up an activity that requires some stamina and energy that you can manage, like knitting or playing a musical instrument.
- If you speak to your doctor, you may be able to get a discount at the gym through the National Health Service.
- If you are overweight, then weigh yourself and aim to lose five to ten per cent of your body weight, because this can significantly improve your health.

Carotid or other artery disease

The carotid artery is the main artery that you can feel on both sides of your neck when you check your pulse there. It is a large artery that supplies blood to the brain, and as it rises up through the neck it branches off to supply all of the different sections of the brain. However, when fatty plaque levels build up in a person's body, one of the places it tends to deposit is on the carotid artery in the neck. The artery can become partially blocked with a large clot, but this can last for years without any symptoms or with very subtle symptoms. The large clot sometimes breaks down every so often to let off tiny clots that lodge in the brain, causing mini-strokes or dementia. This is why, in some cases after a stroke, a carotid Doppler scan is done to see how much blockage there is in the carotid artery. The artery can be almost totally blocked in some cases. If a person is healthy enough to undergo major surgery, then a 'carotid endarterectomy' may be done, which is where the artery is opened up and the clot removed. It is a complex procedure with complications, which is why it may only be offered to those people who are most symptomatic and with larger blockages of the artery.

Other arteries can become blocked by atheroma, such as the vessels in the legs. This leads to pain on exercise; for example, walking up a hill may cause sharp stabbing pains in the legs. When this damage to the leg vessels becomes worse, the pain can occur even at rest. If you have leg pains like this, then it is important to see a doctor because you may need ultrasound scans of the leg arteries and treatment.

Irregular heart beat

Some people have an abnormally fast irregular heart beat, which may be caused by heart disease as well as other medical conditions such as thyroid dysfunction and high alcohol intake. The heart beats so quickly and irregularly that clots form in the heart itself and can be thrown out into the bloodstream, resulting in strokes or heart attacks. People with atrial fibrillation can be given medication to slow down their heart rate, make the heart rate regular, and make the blood thinner so that clots don't form so easily.

Alcohol

You may be thinking, 'I thought alcohol was good for me!' Red wine is thought to make your risk lower because it contains anti-oxidants, which prevent damage to vessel walls, and it increases levels of 'good' cholesterol (HDL). Alcohol in moderation is safe, but drinking over the recommended daily amounts can result in heart attacks, irregular heart beats, liver disease, high blood pressure, high cholesterol, central obesity and many other conditions that either contribute to developing a stroke or make recovery after a stroke much less likely.

Cutting down alcohol

The recommended daily consumption of alcohol is three to four units of alcohol for men, and two to three units for women. One unit of alcohol is half a pint of normal strength lager, a small glass of wine, or a measure of spirits. It is easy to be on the cusp of the recommended daily amount and feel like this is OK, but if you have other risk factors then reducing your alcohol intake can have positive effects on your heart, blood vessels and liver. It is more and more common for young people to start drinking heavily at a young age, socially, and to carry on this habit beyond their teenage years and early twenties, leading to liver disease, irregular heart beats, obesity and general poor health.

Although alcohol has been shown to be good for you in moderation, this can easily be overstepped. I have met many people who shared a bottle of wine with their partner at home every evening and ended up with an irregular heart beat or became dangerously overweight, and nowadays this happens at younger and younger ages. Reducing your alcohol intake requires you first to count the number of units you are having. If you know you are over the limit, then try to be aware of how much you need to reduce your intake. Look at your pattern of drinking – do you drink socially or on your own? Drinking on your own is often a sign of strain and stress, and it can easily spiral out of control without someone to support you. Tell people who drink with you that you are trying to cut down, and try to take time over each individual drink. Have a non-alcoholic drink in between your alcoholic ones. Tell your family and friends that you are trying to cut down so that they can support you. There are support groups and counsellors available to speak to you if you are worried about your alcohol intake. Ask your doctor if you feel like you need help cutting down.

11

Social support after stroke

Care packages after a stroke

After having a stroke, a decision needs to be made about who will care for you, if this is needed. The multidisciplinary team will decide on what care you will need initially after a stroke, and start to arrange this from hospital. A hospital social worker may hand this over to the community social worker. A care manager or social worker is allocated to each person after a stroke and comes to make an assessment of his or her needs, as well as an assessment of finances. The care manager or social worker may arrange for carers to come in up to three times a day to help you to wash, dress, eat, or to help with shopping or giving medications. Sometimes a district nurse may be arranged to change any dressings, give medications and do other tasks of this nature. If you are unable to prepare food, then meals on wheels may be provided.

However, in some cases, people need full-time care, and this means they go to a specialist care home or residential home to receive 24 hour care, which provides all of the above services in a place where people with similar needs also reside.

If you do not have these provisions you can contact your local authority to ask for input from a social worker. Whether you pay for services or not depends on your financial situation. Some services are provided by the social services department, and some may be provided by voluntary organizations or charities. It is important to be clear on what needs you have so that the assessment is appropriate. Ask someone to speak on your behalf or help you to communicate with the social services department if communication is difficult for you. Keep a record of who you talk to and be sure to keep all of the paperwork in a safe place.

Financial assistance

In the UK various organizations can help provide financial assistance to people who have had a stroke and their carers. In addition, many charities and foundations reserve special funds for people in need, and it is worth finding out more about how to get these funds from associations such as The Stroke Association and Different Strokes. (See Useful contacts at the end of this book.)

The Government provides specific benefits schemes for people with disability or on low incomes. Below are some details about financial benefits you should be aware of.

State pension

If you are a woman aged 60 years or a man aged 65 years who made National Insurance Contributions while you were working, then you are entitled to a state pension. If you are divorced or widowed, then you may get a pension or pension increase if you can provide your former partner's financial records.

Pension credit

People on lower incomes may be entitled to guarantee credit, and those on slightly higher incomes may be entitled to a savings credit. If you are disabled, a carer, or receiving housing benefits, you may receive more credit depending on how much money you have saved.

Both of these credits ensure that you receive a minumum weekly income, the amount of which is set by the Government. Contact the Pension Credit Line (telephone: 0800 99 12 34) to apply.

Council Tax Benefit

If you are a pensioner with less than £16,000 in savings or get guarantee credit, then you do not need to pay Council Tax.

If you live alone you should get 25 per cent off your Council Tax bill, and if you are disabled you should also get a discount. If your house is unoccupied, then you should not be paying Council Tax at all. Contact your local authority to get the forms to ensure that you are not paying too much.

Housing benefits

If you are a pensioner with less than £16,000 in savings and pay rent, and if you do not live with a close relative, then you may be entitled to housing benefits. Call the Housing and Council Tax Benefit section of your local council or visit the Department for Work and Pensions website (<http://www.dwp.gov.uk/>).

Heating costs

If you are aged 60 to 79 years and receive pension credit, then you are entitled to a winter fuel payment of £200. If you are over 80 years you get around £300 to help with heating costs. In cold weather extra payments may be made. If you are on a low income, then let your energy supplier know because they may offer free insulation and other services. Visit the Winter Fuel Payments website (<www.thepensionservice.gov.uk/winterfuel>) or make contact by telephone (08459 15 15 15, or 0845 601 5613 for textphone users).

Help with health care costs

If you are aged over 60 years you are entitled to free NHS (National Health Service) prescriptions and sight tests. NHS hearing aids are also available on free loan. You might also be eligible for free chiropody if you have a clinical need. You are automatically entitled to help with health costs if you receive guarantee credit, which means free NHS dental check ups and treatment, sight tests and vouchers toward the cost of glasses or contact lenses, and repayment of necessary travel costs to hospital and back for NHS treatment. You can also obtain discounts if you have less than £16,000 in savings. You should complete a HC11 claim form, which you can get from your doctor, any hospital, or the post office.

Attendance allowance

Attendance allowance is extra income for people with health problems and who require carers. This applies for anyone over 65 with a physical or mental disability, or who is terminally ill. You must be receiving some sort of care and must have required this help for six months before applying for the allowance (unless you are terminally ill, in which case you can apply straight away). Visit the Directgov website (<http://www.direct .gov.uk/en/index.htm>) for more information.

Disability living allowance

If you have any personal care need or physical disability, then you should apply for this. Visit the Directgov website (<http:// www.direct.gov.uk/en/index.htm>) for more information.

Carer's allowance

If you are a carer and cannot work full-time because of your role as a carer, then you may be entitled to carer's allowance. As well as this, if you are a carer under pension age, you should also receive National Insurance credits toward your pension.

The person you care for has to be receiving disability living allowance or attendance allowance, and you must be spending at least 35 hours per week caring for that person. You must earn no more than £95 per week after income tax. If you receive the state pension or other benefits, you may not be entitled to carer's allowance. Visit the Directgov website (<http://www .direct.gov.uk/en/index.htm>) for more information.

The social fund

This allowance is for when you need to make a large payment for a funeral, or housing repairs, or if you are under financial pressure for other reasons. You can apply if you receive other benefits.

Check the Job Centre or visit the Directgov website (<http:// www.direct.gov.uk/en/index.htm>) for more information.

Other concessions

Other concessions you may be entitled to include the following:

- *Free off-peak bus travel.* If you are over 60 you should be able to get a free bus pass.
- *Free TV licence.* If you are over 75 then the licence is free, and you get 50 per cent off if you are registered blind.
- *Orange Badge scheme.* If you apply to your local authority, you can get a disabled badge for display in your car for reduced fare parking and free parking.
- *London's Freedom Pass.* If you are over 60 or if you are disabled, you can travel for free on the underground and buses if you apply for a Freedom Pass.

Respite care

Sometimes a carer and a person who has had a stroke may need a break from each other, or a break to go away individually. Respite care can be provided by day centres. People can go there for a day or more if they will not have their usual care package at home for any reason. Usually, activities are organized and it is a nice experience. Sometimes, carers in place of the usual care package can be arranged instead. Ask your doctor or social worker about organizing respite care.

If you have problems with your carers ...

Sadly, some people do not get on well with their carers or, in a few cases, are even abused by them. If you have any concerns about how your carers look after you, or how they make you feel, do get in touch with Age Concern (Freephone: 0800 00 99 66) or consult your doctor.

12

Stroke services for young people

Strokes in children

Although the majority of strokes occur in people over the age of 60, there are still many who have strokes at ages under 60, and a small number of cases occur in childhood and adolescence. Roughly one in ten strokes occur in people under 30. Because stroke services tend to be aimed at older people, it can be doubly difficult for a younger person with a stroke to fit into the services available.

Young children have strokes that present in the same way as adults, with speech problems, visual disturbances and weakness on one side of the body, but the cause is usually a complex medical condition, rather than long-term damage to blood vessels. Investigations are similar to those in adults but they are carried out in a children's hospital. The same team members are involved but they tend to be specialists in children's needs after a stroke, and include speech and language therapists, physiotherapists and occupational therapists tailored to children. The techniques used in children are similar to those used in adults, with more emphasis on practising play techniques and social interaction with other children. Development in a child is emphasized, so any rehabilitation aims at what other children of the same age can do. For example, if a child has weakness of the right arm and right leg, depending on their age they may be at crawling, walking, running, hopping or skipping stage, and the aim is for them to be able to do the highest complexity of task for their age. If there is a physical impairment, the occupational therapist and physiotherapist work with the child to teach him or her ways to overcome the disability with physical techniques or with physical aids. The team works closely with the family and the school, and after discharge from the hospital a community paediatrician (children's doctor) and community multidisciplinary team will continue to look after the child's social, psychological and physical needs. Getting back to school may take time, and it is important to keep the child in touch with friends during that time and work closely with the local education authority to make sure that the child does return to school at the right time.

Long-term treatment may be necessary in some children, depending on the cause of the stroke. In cases in which a clot caused the stroke, for example, the child may have to take blood-thinning agents. In children with sickle-cell disease who have strokes, blood transfusions can reduce the risk for another stroke.

Strokes in young people

In adolescents and young adults, the impact of a stroke can be as devastating as for older people, but is made still worse by lack of services for a particular age group. For example, for obvious reasons a 27-year-old person may not want to attend the same rehabilitation services as a 70-year-old person, because this can feel embarrassing and can impinge on his or her social networks. Charities such as The Stroke Association and Different Strokes (which is specifically aimed at young people) can provide assistance.

Different Strokes is a charity aimed at younger people who have had a stroke, and was established because stroke services for young people were so poor. This charity has created almost 50 exercise groups in the UK for younger people, and provides specialist information about financial benefits for young people, with paper information as well as online resources. The organization can put you in touch with charities that provide financial assistance and help you to fill in the relevant forms. They also advise on how to get help from social services and benefits, and provide detailed information packs on getting back to work after a stroke, sex after a stroke, preventing further strokes, and more. One of their greatest resources is the interactive message board for people to discuss their own situations and stories, and share experiences to help others.

The Stroke Association is also worth contacting for financial aid, education and assistance. National organizations such as these can pinpoint local services for young people. Their websites are comprehensive, and the person on the other end of the phone is always experienced and helpful.

The medicines used in stroke for young people are the same as those in adults but sometimes at lower doses, and rehabilitation aims at getting the person back to their usual level of functioning, socializing and education.

Conclusion

The fear of having a stroke or of a loved one having a stroke can be overwhelming, and after a stroke the worries that overcome you and your family are understandable because the future is unpredictable and the challenges that a stroke pose may be the greatest emotional and physical ones that you will ever experience. However, I hope that by reading this book you will better understand some of what is going on in your body before, during and after a stroke, and that you will be able to modify your lifestyle and your attitude to recovery after a stroke using your new knowledge about every aspect of treatment and prevention. If you are a family member, partner, or friend of someone who has had a stroke, then you should now be equipped with facts that may help you to change your loved one's attitude to his or her health if necessary, and to work alongside them to improve both your health and theirs.

There are two points I wanted to emphasize when I wrote this book.

- It is never too late to change your lifestyle and your health for the better, even after a stroke.
- After a stroke it is possible to live a full life, if you maintain a positive attitude toward rehabilitation.

I hope these points and more have come across, and I wish you all the best on your continuing journey.

Useful contacts

Acquire see **Trust-Ed**

Afasic
Second Floor
20 Bowling Green Lane
London EC1R 0BD
Tel.: 020 7490 9410 (general
enquiries); 0845 355 5577 (helpline,
10.30 a.m. to 2.30 p.m., Monday to
Friday)
Website: www.afasic.org.uk

For children and young people with
speech problems after a stroke.

Age Concern England
Astral House
1268 London Road
London SW16 4ER
Helpline: 0800 00 99 66 (free)
Website: www.ageconcern.org.uk

British Pain Society (formerly the
Pain Society)
Third Floor, Churchill House
35 Red Lion Square
London WC1R 4SG
Tel.: 020 7269 7840
Website: www.britishpainsociety.org

A membership organization of
medical professionals engaged in
the diagnosis and treatment of
pain, and pain research for the
benefit of patients.

Carer's Allowance Unit see
**Department for Work and
Pensions**

Central Pain Syndrome Alliance
Website: www.centralpain.org

An international internet resource
to bring together people around
the world who share a common
bond of chronic neuropathic pain
(Central Pain). Provides links to
other similar websites worldwide.

Chest, Heart & Stroke Scotland
65 North Castle Street
Edinburgh EH2 3LT
Advice line: 0845 077 6000
Website: www.chss.org.uk

Child Brain Injury Trust
Unit 1, The Great Barn
Baynards Green Farm
Bicester
Oxon OX27 7SG
Tel.: 01869 341075; 0845 601 4939
(helpline)
Website: www.cbituk.org

Connect
16–18 Marshalsea Road
London SE1 1HL
Tel.: 020 7367 0840
Website: www.ukconnect.org

Provides services to people with
aphasia (communication disability)
after a stroke.

**Department for Children, Schools
and Families**
Website: www.dcsf.gov.uk/index.
htm or
www.direct.gov.uk/en/Parents/
Schoolslearninganddevelopment/
SpecialEducationNeeds

This government organization
(formerly the **Department for
Education and Skills**) provides
advice for parents and teachers of
children with special education
needs.

Department for Work and Pensions (DWP)
Public Enquiry Office: tel.: 020 7712 2171; fax: 020 7712 2386
Carer's Allowance Unit is part of the DWP; tel.: 01772 899 729 or 01253 85 61 23
Disability Benefits Enquiry Line: 0800 88 22 00
Website: www.dwp.gov.uk/lifeevent/famchild/index.asp

Provides information on a range of benefits and services for families.

Different Strokes
Information Officer
9 Canon Harnett Court
Wolverton Mill
Milton Keynes MK12 5NF
Helpline: 0845 130 7172
Website: www.differentstrokes.co.uk

For younger people who have had a stroke.

Disability Alliance
Universal House
88–94 Wentworth Street
London E1 7SA
Tel.: 020 7247 8776
Website: www.disabilityalliance.org

Provides information and advice to disabled people and their families about entitlement to social security benefits and services.

Disability Benefits Enquiry Line
see **Department for Work and Pensions**

The Government's UK website
provides access to all its public services and information: www.direct.gov.uk/en/index.htm

HemiHelp
Camelford House
89 Albert Embankment
London SE1 7TP
Tel.: 0845 120 3713
Helpline: 0845 123 2372 (10 a.m. to 1 p.m., Monday to Friday, termtime).
Website: www.hemihelp.org.uk

Provides information and support for children with hemiplegia and their families.

InterAct Reading Service
Spur C, Fourth Floor
Charles House
375 Kensington High Street
London W14 8QH
Tel.: 020 7471 6789
Website: www.interactreading.org

Provides a professional, live, interactive reading service for stroke patients in hospitals and stroke clubs.

Northern Ireland Chest, Heart & Stroke
21 Dublin Road
Belfast BT2 7HB
Tel.: 028 9032 0184
Helpline: 08457 697 299
Website: www.nichsa.com

Provides help and rehabilitation for stroke and cardiac patients and their carers through a network of clubs.

Pain Concern
PO Box 13256
Haddington
East Lothian EH41 4YD
Listening Ear helpline: 01620 822 572 (9 a.m. to 5 p.m., Monday to Friday: a chance to talk to another person experiencing pain)

Website: www.painconcern.org.uk

Supports those experiencing chronic pain and their carers with a range of self-help leaflets, books and audiotapes; the quarterly *Pain Matters* includes updates on latest developments in pain management and how to cope. There are also links to other websites.

Speakability
1 Royal Street
London SE1 7LL
Tel.: 020 7261 9572
Helpline: 0808 808 9572
Website: www.speakability.org.uk

Provides support and advice for people through publications and local network groups, and training for health care professionals. It promotes self-empowerment among people with aphasia.

Speakeasy
Market Chambers
5 Market Place
Ramsbottom
Bury BL0 9AJ
Tel: 01706 825802
Website: www.buryspeakeasy.org.uk

Offers support and advice for people with aphasia, mainly in the north-west of England, to maintain the progress made with speech therapy after regular therapy comes to an end.

Stroke Association
Stroke Information Service
240 City Road
London EC1V 2PR.
Helpline: 0845 3033 100 (9 a.m. to 5 p.m., Monday to Friday; local rate within UK).

Website: www.stroke.org.uk

The Stroke Association is solely concerned with combating instances of stroke in people of all ages. It funds research into prevention, treatment and better methods of rehabilitation, and assists families and carers through its Rehabilitation and Support Services, providing leaflets and a quarterly journal, *Stroke News*.

Trust-Ed (formerly **Acquire**)
PO Box 6016
Keyworth
Nottingham NG12 5RP
Website: www.trust-ed.org

Provides educational services for young people with acquired brain injury.

United Kingdom Acquired Brain Injury Forum (UKABIF)
PO Box 355
Plymouth PL3 4WD
Tel.: 01752 601318
Website: www.ukabif.org.uk

A coalition of organizations and individuals that seeks to promote understanding of all aspects of acquired brain injury, including that caused by strokes, and to provide information to promote the interests of brain-injured people and their families and carers.

UK College of Hydrotherapy
515 Hagley Road
Birmingham B66 4AX
Tel.: 0121 429 9191
Physiotherapists and naturopaths supervise warm-water exercise, often a useful adjunct to other treatment.

Index